Bioceramic Materials in Clinical Endodontics

Saulius Drukteinis • Josette Camilleri
Editors

Bioceramic Materials in Clinical Endodontics

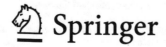

Editors
Saulius Drukteinis
Institute of Dentistry
Vilnius University
Vilnius
Lithuania

Josette Camilleri
Edgbaston
University of Birmingham
Birmingham
UK

ISBN 978-3-030-58172-5   ISBN 978-3-030-58170-1   (eBook)
https://doi.org/10.1007/978-3-030-58170-1

This Springer imprint is published by the registered company Springer Nature Switzerland AG
The registered company address is: Gewerbestrasse 11, 6330 Cham, Switzerland

Preface

The introduction of modified hydraulic calcium silicate-based materials has changed the standards and strategies of endodontics. These new materials and the techniques developed for their use in clinical practice have been extensively investigated in in vitro and in vivo studies and have shown similar or superior results compared to the conventional materials and techniques.

This book describes a classification for the hydraulic calcium silicate-based materials based on materials chemistry and focuses on the newest currently available on the market. Classic, modified or new techniques used in modern endodontics are presented and reviewed.

The first two chapters provide a review and a classification, characterisation and basic understanding of modern hydraulic calcium silicate-based materials and analyse their physical, chemical and biological properties. The remaining clinical chapters of the book address the application of these materials in daily clinical practice. Chapter 3 is dedicated to the current materials and techniques used in vital pulp therapy, while Chap. 4 reviews modern concepts and strategies in regenerative endodontics. Chapter 5 focuses on the most established hydraulic calcium silicate-based sealers and root canal obturation techniques, used in conjunction with these materials. Chapter 6 focuses on the materials for the management of endodontic complications as well as management methods and techniques. Finally, the last chapter reviews hydraulic calcium silicate-based materials and techniques for the treatment of permanent teeth in paediatric patients.

Vilnius, Lithuania   Saulius Drukteinis
Birmingham, UK   Josette Camilleri

Acknowledgements

We would like to acknowledge Springer International Publishing for giving us the opportunity to edit this textbook on Bioceramic Materials in Clinical Endodontics. A special thanks go to Dr. Markus Bartels, who was responsible for offering us this project and to project coordinators Narendran Natarajan and Deepika Devan, who were managing the whole writing-editing-publishing process.

We are indebted to the following collaborators for their hard work and invaluable contributions to make this book possible: Stéphane Simon, Kerstin M. Galler, Matthias Widbiller, Luc C. Martens, Sivaprakash Rajasekharan and other colleagues who allow us the privilege of sharing their images in courtesy. Thank you very much! We especially want to acknowledge Mr. Rousselos Aravantinos for his vast input with composing and editing the figures. We would also like to thank our families, friends and colleagues for their encouragement, assistance and support that allowed us to progress in our professional lives.

Contents

Current Classification of Bioceramic Materials in Endodontics

Josette Camilleri

1 Introduction

In the last few decades, a lot of changes have been introduced in endodontics. The most important ones are the introduction of procedures under magnification and accentuated light that has enabled better visualization, the use of ultrasonics and the introduction of mineral trioxide aggregate (MTA) for various procedures in endodontics.

There has been and there still is a lot of confusion with the importance of using mineral trioxide aggregate in clinical endodontics and why this material is so popular. MTA is a radiopacified Portland cement which in turn is a construction material that has been patented for use in clinical dentistry specifically for root-end filling and perforation repair procedures [1–4]. The main interest for the introduction of MTA for these specific procedures was the hydraulic properties of the Portland cement. This material is well researched in the construction industry, and it has been shown to improve its physical properties in the presence of water [5–7]. The other feature of Portland cement that makes it important in endodontic procedures is its hydration reaction. When Portland cement is mixed with water the components, which are tricalcium and dicalcium silicate and

tricalcium aluminate, undergo a hydration reaction forming calcium silicate hydrate and calcium hydroxide from the silicate reaction and ettringite and monosulphate from the interaction of the aluminate in the presence of calcium sulphate that is added to the cement by the manufacturer. The formation of calcium hydroxide makes the use of Portland cement multifaceted as it can be used for all procedures where calcium hydroxide is employed, including vital pulp procedures. Due to this, the most important features of MTA can be noted as being its specific chemistry, the hydration and hydraulic properties. It has been suggested that MTA should be classified as a hydraulic calcium silicate cement [8] as this takes into consideration both its specific chemistry and the hydraulic properties which make it quite unique in endodontics. Since the expiry of the patent restrictions, several materials with a similar chemistry have been introduced in clinical practice. These materials and the nomenclature will be discussed.

2 Classification of Hydraulic Cements

The hydraulic cements available in clinical practice are no longer simple mixtures of Portland cement and bismuth oxide radiopacifier, mixed with water. There have been significant material modifications and thus a classification is

J. Camilleri (✉)
University of Birmingham, Birmingham, UK
e-mail: J.Camilleri@bham.ac.uk

© Springer Nature Switzerland AG 2021
S. Drukteinis, J. Camilleri (eds.), *Bioceramic Materials in Clinical Endodontics*,
https://doi.org/10.1007/978-3-030-58170-1_1

necessary [9]. Hydraulic cements can be classified depending on use. This classification is shown in Table 1 [9]. It is helpful for clinicians as it guides the material users on the environment in which it has been developed for and the specific standard that the material complies to.

A more robust classification is based on the material chemistry [9]. The original MTA formulation was based on radiopacified Portland cement mixed with water. Figure 1 shows the different components of such systems and this can help with classifying the materials based on their chemistry. The main four components of hydraulic cement systems are the cement, radiopacifier, the vehicle and the additives. Variations to these components create the different types of hydraulic cements.

To date there are five types of hydraulic calcium silicate cements as indicated in Table 2. The different types have been created with specific aims to overcome the shortcomings of the original MTA formulation. The main sub-classification is the distinction between the Portland cement types and the ones whose main cementitious component is synthetic as are the tricalcium silicate–based materials. The radiopacifier is not given a separate classification, since although it impacts on certain material characteristics, it does not change the cement chemistry substantially. The other subdivisions are based on the presence or absence of additives and whether the materials are mixed with water or are delivered in suspension and they interact with the liquid present in the environment in order to set. This classification is described in detail in a recent publication [9].

The Type 1 includes all materials based on Portland cement that may or may not be radiopacified, do not include additives and which are

Table 1 Classification of hydraulic cements based on their specific use in endodontology [9]

Location	Specific use
Intra-coronal	Pulp capping materials
	Regenerative endodontic cements
Intra-radicular	Root canal sealers
	Apical plug cements
	Perforation repair cements
Extra-radicular	Root-end filling materials
	Perforation repair cements

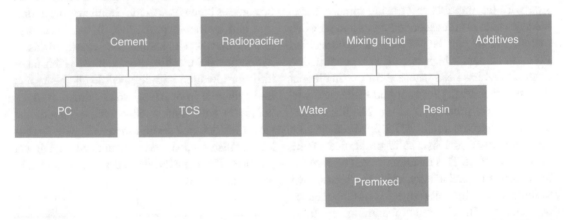

Fig. 1 Diagrammatic representation of hydraulic cements in clinical use showing the main components of the different material types

Table 2 Classification of hydraulic cements based on their chemistry

Type	Cement	Radiopacifier	Additives	Water
1	Portland cement	✔/X	X	✔
2	Portland cement	✔	✔	✔
3	Portland cement	✔	✔	X
4	Tricalcium/Dicalcium silicate	✔	✔	✔
5	Tricalcium/Dicalcium silicate	✔	✔	X

mixed with water. MTA is a Type 1 material with ProRoot MTA (Dentsply, Tulsa, OK, USA) being typical. The unradiopacified Portland cement, which is a medical grade (Medcem, Vienna, Austria), is also a Type 1 cement. Most other brands have additives, thus are classified as Type 2 cements. These additives aim at enhancing the early release of the calcium hydroxide such as the calcium oxide in MTA Angelus (Angelus, Londrina, Brazil) [10], the bioactivity such as additions of hydroxyapatite in the Bio MTA+ by Cerkamed (Cerkamed, Stalowa Wola, Poland) or the mechanical performance and setting time like MM-MTA (Coltene Micro-Mega, Besancon, France) which includes calcium carbonate as filler and calcium chloride as accelerator [11]. The replacement of the water by alternative vehicles are the Type 3 cements. These include Endoseal (Gangwon-do, South Korea) and similar premixed materials. The setting of these cement types depends on the imbibition of fluids from the surroundings. MTA Fillapex is mostly composed of salicylate resin, and TheraCal has a light-curable hydrophilic resin matrix thus it is debatable whether these materials can be classed as hydraulic cements.

The Type 4 (Biodentine, Septodont, Saint-Maur-des-Fosses, France; BioAggregate, BioCeramix inc., Vancouver, Canada) and Type 5 materials (TotalFill, FKG, La Chaux-de-Fonds, Switzerland) are tricalcium silicate–based. The Type 4 materials are mixed with water while the Type 5 are referred to premixed materials. The term premixed is a misnomer since the essential ingredient needed for the hydration is missing. To be premixed, the materials need to have all the components and the setting prohibited by hydration blockers which are not the case with the Type 5 materials.

The primary goal of introducing the tricalcium silicate–based materials was the elimination of the Portland cement. The use of alternative cements to the Portland cement has stemmed following concerns with the presence of aluminium and trace elements such as chromium, arsenic and lead in the Portland cement. The use of trical-

cium silicate as an alternative to Portland cement was patented by BioCeramix Inc (Vancouver, Canada), where the aluminium-free formulation of the hydraulic cement is mentioned in their patent application 7553362 in 2006 [12]. The original formulation was BioAggregate (BioCeramix Inc., Vancouver, Canada) which was presented as a powder to liquid formulation thus as Type 4 cement. Later reports indicated the migration and potential toxicity of aluminium in an animal model with traces of it found in the serum [13] and causing oxidative stress in the brain [14]. Another concern with the use of Portland cement–based cements is the trace elements at levels higher than the ISO standard for water-based cements [15]. The standard only specifies the levels of acid-extractable arsenic for zinc phosphate and polycarboxylate cements and lead for the same and for glass-ionomer cements. The chromium levels were also shown to be elevated. Although the acid-extractable arsenic and lead were higher than the ISO norms [16–18] with some brands showing levels higher than others [19–22], the leachate showed only minimal amounts of heavy elements [18, 23]. As for the aluminium, the trace heavy metals were detected in the brain and kidney of test animals [24], thus can be a cause of concern.

Besides replacing the Portland cement, both the BioCeramix Inc. [25, 26] and the Septodont patents [27, 28] specify the use of additives to enhance the material properties. In the BioCeramix Inc. patents [12, 25, 26], calcium phosphate monobasic is added while in the Septodont ones [27, 28], the properties are modified by the addition of calcium carbonate, a water-soluble polymer and calcium chloride. For both material types, the radiopacifier is an alternative to bismuth oxide.

The premixed versions of the BioCeramix Inc. materials were patented later [29]. These materials are now marketed as EndoSequence BC (Brasseler, Savannah AU, USA), TotalFill (FKG, La Chaux-de-Fonds, Switzerland) and iRoot (BioCeramix Inc., Vancouver, Canada). Although they have different labels they are the same materials.

3   Bioceramics and Hydraulic Calcium Silicate Cements

There is some confusion with which materials can be classed as bioceramics. Bioceramics is the broader definition of all hydraulic calcium silicate cements. However, the first paper to mention the bioceramics in endodontics refers to BioAggregate (BioCeramix Inc, Vancouver, Canada) [30]. The patent also refers to this invention as a bioceramic [12], and this terminology clearly refers to a new type of material that is tricalcium silicate–based indicating the change in the cement type and the lack of aluminium in its composition. The first papers describing the clin-

ical use of bioceramics refer to the same materials types [31, 32]. It can thus be concluded that the new terminology was created to distinguish the tricalcium silicate–based cements from the ones that are Portland cement–based thus indicating that the bioceramics are purer and bioactive.

4   Clinical Presentation

Besides showing distinct chemistries, the hydraulic calcium silicate–based cements are also provided in a variety of presentations as shown in Fig. 2. This enhances the material mixing and delivery methods in clinical practice.

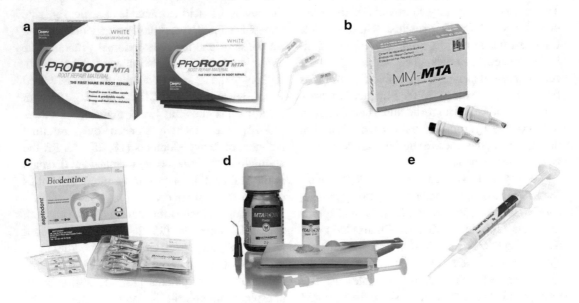

Fig. 2 Different clinical presentations of hydraulic calcium silicate cements (**a**) ProRoot MTA as powder to liquid, (**b**) MM-MTA in capsule and gun, (**c**) Biodentine also in capsule but no gun or syringe delivery, (**d**) MTA Flow which is also a powder and liquid but has a disposable syringe for ease of material delivery and (**e**) TotalFill BC as premixed materials in syringes

5 Conclusions

Bioceramics in endodontics are the materials that are composed of tricalcium silicate–based cement synthesized from lab-grade chemicals and not including aluminium in their composition. These are classified as Types 4 and 5 hydraulic calcium silicate cements and have specific chemistries and material properties.

References

1. Torabinejad M, White JD. Tooth filling material and method of use. Patent number: 5415547; 1993.
2. Torabinejad M, White JD. Tooth filling material and method of use. Patent number: 5769638; 1995.
3. Primus C. Dental material. Publication number: 20030159618; 2002.
4. Primus C. Dental material. Patent number: 7892342; 2009.
5. Taylor HFW. Cement chemistry. London: Thomas Telford; 1997. p. 113–225.
6. Odler I. Hydration, setting and hardening of Portland cement. In: Lea's chemistry of cement and concrete. London: Arnold; 1998. p. 241–84.
7. Moir GK. Cements. In: Newman J, Choo BS, editors. Advanced concrete technology: constituent materials. Oxford: Elsevier Butterworth Heinemann; 2003. p. 3–45.
8. Darvell BW, Wu RC. "MTA"—an hydraulic silicate cement: review update and setting reaction. Dent Mater. 2011;27(5):407–22.
9. Camilleri J. Classification of hydraulic cements used in Dentistry. Frontiers in Dental Medicine - Dental Materials 2020; https://doi.org/10.3389/fdmed.2020.00009
10. Camilleri J, Sorrentino F, Damidot D. Investigation of the hydration and bioactivity of radiopacified tricalcium silicate cement, biodentine and MTA angelus. Dent Mater. 2013;29(5):580–93.
11. Khalil I, Naaman A, Camilleri J. Investigation of a novel mechanically mixed mineral trioxide aggregate (MM-MTA(™)). Int Endod J. 2015;48(8):757–67.
12. Lu D, Zhou S. High strength biological cement composition and using the same. Patent number: 7553362; 2006.
13. Demirkaya K, Can Demirdögen B, Öncel Torun Z, Erdem O, Çetinkaya S, Akay C. In vivo evaluation of the effects of hydraulic calcium silicate dental cements on plasma and liver aluminium levels in rats. Eur J Oral Sci. 2016;124(1):75–81.
14. Demirkaya K, Demirdögen BC, Torun ZÖ, Erdem O, Çırak E, Tunca YM. Brain aluminium accumulation and oxidative stress in the presence of calcium silicate dental cements. Hum Exp Toxicol. 2017;36(10):1071–80.
15. International Standards Organization. Dentistry-water-based cements—Part 1: Powder/liquid acid-base cements. ISO 9917-1: 2007; 2007.
16. Chang SW, Shon WJ, Lee W, Kum KY, Baek SH, Bae KS. Analysis of heavy metal contents in gray and white MTA and 2 kinds of Portland cement: a preliminary study. Oral Surg Oral Med Oral Pathol Oral Radiol Endod. 2010;109(4):642–6.
17. Schembri M, Peplow G, Camilleri J. Analyses of heavy metals in mineral trioxide aggregate and Portland cement. J Endod. 2010;36(7):1210–5.
18. Camilleri J, Kralj P, Veber M, Sinagra E. Characterization and analyses of acid-extractable and leached trace elements in dental cements. Int Endod J. 2012;45(8):737–43.
19. Monteiro Bramante C, Demarchi AC, de Moraes IG, Bernadineli N, Garcia RB, Spångberg LS, Duarte MA. Presence of arsenic in different types of MTA and white and gray Portland cement. Oral Surg Oral Med Oral Pathol Oral Radiol Endod. 2008;106(6):909–13.
20. De-Deus G, de Souza MC, Sergio Fidel RA, Fidel SR, de Campos RC, Luna AS. Negligible expression of arsenic in some commercially available brands of Portland cement and mineral trioxide aggregate. J Endod. 2009;35(6):887–90. https://doi.org/10.1016/j.joen.2009.03.003.
21. Chang SW, Baek SH, Yang HC, Seo DG, Hong ST, Han SH, Lee Y, Gu Y, Kwon HB, Lee W, Bae KS, Kum KY. Heavy metal analysis of ortho MTA and ProRoot MTA. J Endod. 2011;37(12):1673–6.
22. Kum KY, Zhu Q, Safavi K, Gu Y, Bae KS, Chang SW. Analysis of six heavy metals in Ortho mineral trioxide aggregate and ProRoot mineral trioxide aggregate by inductively coupled plasma-optical emission spectrometry. Aust Endod J. 2013;39(3):126–30.
23. Duarte MA, De Oliveira Demarchi AC, Yamashita JC, Kuga MC, De Campos Fraga S. Arsenic release provided by MTA and Portland cement. Oral Surg Oral Med Oral Pathol Oral Radiol Endod. 2005;99(5):648–50.
24. Simsek N, Bulut ET, Ahmetoğlu F, Alan H. Determination of trace elements in rat organs implanted with endodontic repair materials by ICP-MS. J Mater Sci Mater Med. 2016;27(3):46.
25. Lu D, Zhou S. Hydraulic cement compositions and methods of making and using the same. Patent number: 7575628; 2006.
26. Lu D, Zhou S. Hydraulic cement compositions and methods of making and using the same. Patent number: 8343271; 2009.

27. Bergaya B, Bottero JY, Bottero MJ, Franquin JC, LeBlanc D, Marie O, Nonat A, Sauvaget C. Preparation for producing a material used to restore a mineralised substance, particularly in the dental field. Patent number: 7819663; 2003.
28. Richard G, Marie O, Bafounguissa L. Wear resistant dental composition. Patent number: 9427380; 2012.
29. Yang Q, Lu D. Premixed biological hydraulic cement paste composition and using the same. Patent number: 8475811; 2008.
30. De-Deus G, Canabarro A, Alves G, Linhares A, Senne MI, Granjeiro JM. Optimal cytocompatibility of a bioceramic nanoparticulate cement in primary human mesenchymal cells. J Endod. 2009;35(10):1387–90.
31. Koch KA, Brave DG, Nasseh AA. Bioceramic technology: closing the endo-restorative circle, Part I. Dent Today. 2010;29(2):100–5.
32. Koch KA, Brave GD, Nasseh AA. Bioceramic technology: closing the endo-restorative circle, part 2. Dent Today. 2010;29(3):98, 100, 102–5.

Characterization and Properties of Bioceramic Materials for Endodontics

Josette Camilleri

1 Introduction

The bioceramics are a specific class of endodontic materials that are composed primarily of synthetic tricalcium silicate that is manufactured under strict laboratory conditions from lab-grade raw materials and are aluminium-free [1]. These material types include a radiopacifier and additives to enhance their properties. They can be either water-based (Type 4) or referred to as premixed (Type 5) where the powders are suspended in an alternative vehicle, and these materials set when in contact with the moist dental tissues. The material properties for each specific use vary. The properties of these materials used coronally, intra-radicularly and extra-radicularly will be discussed. For each use, the material chemistry, physical and mechanical properties, biological and antimicrobial characteristics, the clinical use and clinical interactions will be reviewed. The clinical success rates for each material types will also be discussed.

2 Coronal Use

The coronal use of hydraulic calcium silicate cements includes their use for pulp preservation procedures which encompasses indirect, direct pulp therapy and pulpotomy of permanent teeth. Furthermore, they are also used for apexogenesis procedures in immature permanent teeth and as a barrier material in regenerative endodontic procedures.

Both the Type 4 and Type 5 cements are suitable for coronal use. However, the premixed materials do not seem to have a history of being used for these procedures. This could be due to the limited amount of fluids available in pulp protection procedures and also the long setting time, which would preclude or complicate the clinical technique. The most important feature necessary for the coronal use of hydraulic calcium silicate–based cements is the calcium ion release, which although has been implicated with barrier formation and enhanced biological properties seems to play a major role in antimicrobial characteristics [2].

2.1 Chemical, Physical and Mechanical Properties

Setting time, adequate surface hardness and colour stability are important characteristics for materials used for vital pulp therapy. These

J. Camilleri (✉)
University of Birmingham, Birmingham, UK
e-mail: J.Camilleri@bham.ac.uk

© Springer Nature Switzerland AG 2021
S. Drukteinis, J. Camilleri (eds.), *Bioceramic Materials in Clinical Endodontics*,
https://doi.org/10.1007/978-3-030-58170-1_2

characteristics can be achieved by the use of additives and appropriate radiopacifiers.

The only hydraulic water-based material that has been specifically developed to be used for pulp preservation procedures is Biodentine® (Septodont, Saint-Maur-des-Fosses, France). It is a Type 4 material, thus it is mixed with water for the hydration reaction. Tricalcium silicate is the main component. The additives include calcium carbonate, which is added to the powder; calcium chloride and water-soluble polymer make part of the liquid together with the water. The water-soluble polymer enables the use of less water to obtain the same consistency [3–5] and this, together with the calcium carbonate, makes the material stronger [6, 7]. The setting time is controlled with the calcium chloride as has been reported in the literature for MTA and Portland cement [8–10]. The radiopacifier is zirconium oxide; thus it is not implicated in tooth discolouration [11–13].

Biodentine® exhibits a higher initial rate of calcium ion release compared to other similar material types [14, 15]. This is due to the interaction of the calcium carbonate which enhances the reaction rate [6]. The hydration of Biodentine® proceeds well with the limited fluid available diffusing through the tooth to material interface [16].

2.2 Biological Characteristics

The biological characteristics of Biodentine® indicate favourable cell proliferation and alkaline phosphatase activity of human dental pulp cells [17–20] and formation of reactionary and reparative dentine [21] which is essential for all pulp capping and apexogenesis procedures. Biodentine® was also shown to enhance proliferation and odontoblast differentiation of human stem cells [21, 22] indicating its suitability as a barrier material in regenerative endodontic procedures. Other features of Biodentine® include the expression and release of dentine matrix proteins [23], anti-inflammatory potential and induced the pulp regeneration capacity [24].

Furthermore, it enhanced mineralized tissue formation [25–27].

Biodentine® also shows antimicrobial effect [28–31] including its leachate [15]. The calcium ion release has been shown to be important, particularly for the material antimicrobial properties [2].

2.3 Clinical Performance and Material Interactions

Pulp protection materials are placed in contact with dentine and pulp. In turn, they are layered with a restorative material. The material reactivity makes the clinical performance very challenging. The dentine is caries affected dentine rather than sound dentine. Adhesion to caries affected dentine is challenging due to the microbial loading and the specific dentine microstructure. The use of sodium hypochlorite to condition the dentine prior to application of the hydraulic cements enhanced the material bonding to dentine [32]. The hypochlorite also is meant to reduce the microbial load and is recommended by the ESE guidelines [33].

The interaction of Biodentine® with dentine has been shown to be by elemental migration at the tooth to material interface resulting in a mineral infiltration zone in the dentine at the interface [34]. This has been disputed as no exchange of calcium and phosphorus was shown at the interface with the migration of silicon being mostly evident [35] and the deposition of the calcium phosphate in the interfacial zone [36, 37]. Removal of smear layer and whether it improves the material interaction with dentine is also not well researched; however, the use of 17% EDTA applied for 1 min resulted in a tighter interface [35].

The interaction of hydraulic cements with blood has been investigated, and when used for regenerative endodontic procedures, the formation of calcium carbonate has been verified [38]. The other challenge with using hydraulic calcium silicate materials coronally is the tooth restoration, particularly with the water-based materials. Although it has been shown that materials such as Biodentine® are strong enough to be used as temporary filling materials for up to 6 months [39], it is ideal to restore the tooth on the same visit. Material preparation for placement of composite resin restorations makes hydraulic cements weaker as etching results in the destruction of the material microstructure (Fig. 1a) [40]. Bond strengths of composite resin to hydraulic cements have been shown to be weak [41–47] and not durable [48]. A clear space was shown at the tooth to the material interface after etching (Fig. 1b, c). Reducing the etching times resulted in less material destruction, but the

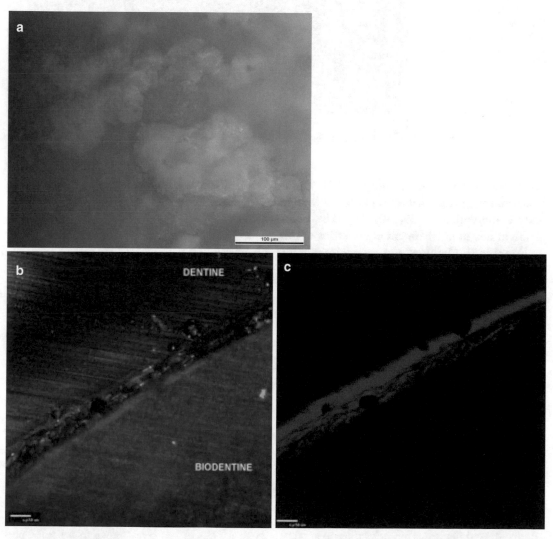

Fig. 1 (a) Light micrograph of Biodentine® surface after application of 37% phosphoric acid showing the surface changes of the material; (b) confocal micrograph of Biodentine® to dentine interface showing the interfacial gap and (c) confocal micrograph enabling the visualiza- tion of the dye that was used to dip the specimens showing the clear interfacial gap between the dentine and Biodentine® after acid etching. (Reprinted with permission from Camilleri 2013 [40])

Fig. 2 Backscatter scanning electron micrograph of Biodentine® to a composite interface showing the good adaptation of the composite resin to the bonding system with cracks in the bonding agent and poor adaptation to the Biodentine® surface. (Reprinted with permission from Camilleri et al., 2014 [16])

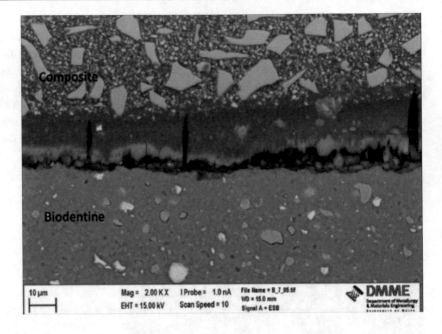

bond strengths were not improved [49]. There is no consensus on whether it is best to wait or restore immediately [39, 50, 51]. The main problem lies in the different chemistries of the hydrophilic Biodentine® and the hydrophobicity of the bonding systems (Fig. 2) [16].

The clinical performance of Biodentine® has been shown to be comparable to MTA [52] with similar dentine bridge formation potential [53]. Higher clinical success rates were shown when using Biodentine® for indirect pulp capping using cone beam computed tomography [54, 55]. The use of Biodentine® has been shown to reverse irreversible pulpitis when used as a dressing over partial or full pulpotomies in permanent teeth [56, 57].

3   Intra-radicular Use

The intra-radicular use of the hydraulic calcium silicate–based materials includes the use as sealers particularly using the single-cone obturation technique and also as an apical plug for immature teeth with an open apex. The materials used intra-radicularly can be both water-based and premixed.

3.1   Chemial, Physical and Mechanical Properties

The hydraulic calcium silicate–based sealer chemistry is quite similar for most brands. The tricalcium silicate is the main cementitious phase with zirconium oxide radiopacifier [58]. Root canal sealers have to comply to ISO specifications—ISO 6976:2012 [59]. The validity of using this standard that has been developed for sealers that do not interact with the media they are placed in is questionable [60]. The testing medium suggested by the standard is water, and the use of physiological solutions has been shown to result in different and contrasting values for solubility, particularly [60]. Thus, the high solubility of hydraulic root canal sealers reported in some studies may be exaggerated [61, 62].

The properties of water-based sealers are quite distinct from those of the premixed sealers. While BioRoot™ RCS (Septodont, Saint-Maur-des-Fosses, France) has been shown to set fully, premixed root canal sealers such as TotalFill® BC Sealer™ (FKG, La Chaux-de-Fonds, Switzerland) do not set when dry [58]. This, questions the validity of drying the root canal completely prior to obturation.

The final setting time of BioRoot™ RCS was shown to be 324 (±1) min which was shorter than that for AH Plus [63]. Most sealers based on hydraulic cement exhibit flow and film thickness that complies with ISO 6976:2012 [59] recommendations. The radiopacity varies from one sealer to the other but most of the sealers showing radiopacity values higher than the 3 mm aluminium thickness [58, 63] specified by the ISO standard.

The calcium ion release also varies between the different sealers. Additives such as calcium phosphate monobasic present in the TotalFill® BC Sealer™ have been shown to reduce the calcium ion release [64]. The TotalFill® BC Sealer™ has a lower calcium ion release than BioRoot™ RCS [58]. Besides the additives that limit the formation of the calcium hydroxide, the hydration of the premixed sealers depends on the water availability in the surroundings and the ion release through diffusion which further delays or restricts the availability of calcium. Microbial challenge has also been shown to reduce the calcium ion release in BioRoot™ RCS [65].

3.2 Biological Characteristics

The biological characteristics of sealers are essential since the sealers are in contact with the periodontal ligament and the bone at the apex. Hydraulic sealers showed a high degree of cell proliferation [66–70]. The cytotoxicity was dose-dependent [71] and the specific material chemistry affects the cell viability, cell attachment and cell migration rates and this was higher for materials releasing higher levels of calcium [72, 73]. The hydraulic sealers also have an osteogenic [73, 74] and an anti-inflammatory effect [74].

Hydraulic calcium silicate–based sealers are antimicrobial [75–77] although the initial antimicrobial properties, particularly in the presence of biofilm, are limited in the early ages [77]. The combined effect of sodium hypochlorite and hydraulic sealers is superior to either in its own; thus showing that when used together, they have a better antimicrobial effect [78].

3.3 Clinical Performance and Material Interactions

The interaction of hydraulic sealers with dentine is similar to what has been reported for pulp preservation materials. Elemental migration at the interface predominantly for the silicon has been demonstrated (Fig. 3a, b) [79, 80].

Since hydraulic sealers are susceptible to changes in their environment, the chemistry of the irrigating solutions is crucial. The irrigating solutions used frequently during root canal therapy are sodium hypochlorite, EDTA and chlorhexidine. The sodium hypochlorite potentiates the antimicrobial effect of hydraulic sealers [78]. The strategy of removal of the smear layer to allow bonding to the exposed collagen works well with resin-based sealers. The mineral interaction reported for the hydraulic sealers [79, 80] cannot occur if calcium chelators are used to remove the mineral and expose the collagen. Furthermore, remnants of calcium chelators such as ethylenediaminetetraacetic acid (EDTA)

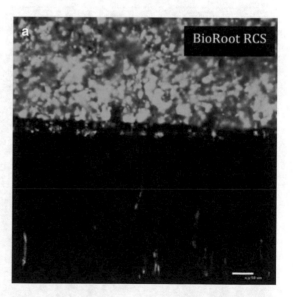

Fig. 3 Sealer interaction with root dentine; (**a**) BioRoot™ RCS in contact with dentine showing both sealer tags and mineral infiltration zone at the interface of the tooth to the material; (**b**) scanning electron micrograph and energy dispersive maps of BioRoot™ RCS sealer in contact with dentine showing the interfacial microstructure and elemental migration across the interface. (Reprinted with permission from Kebudi Benzra et al., 2018 [79])

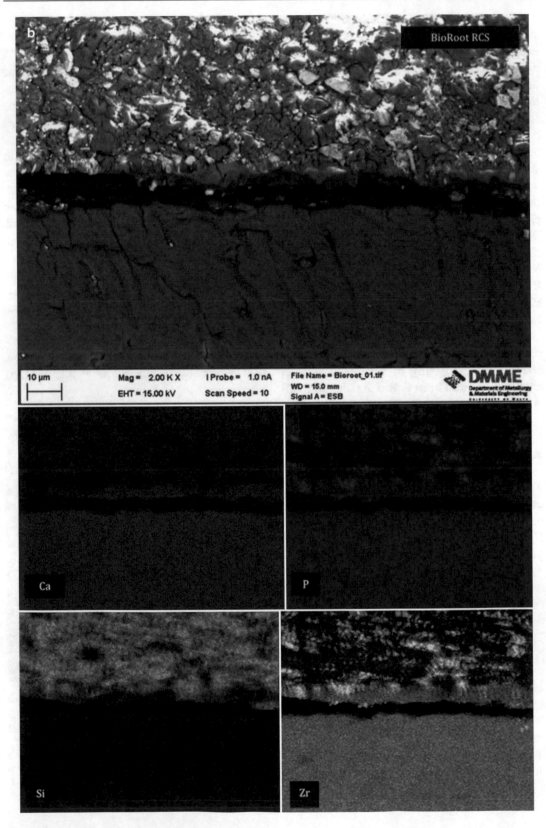

Fig. 3 (continued)

will cause chemical alterations to the sealers [81]. The push-out bond strength of hydraulic sealers was also reduced in the presence of EDTA [82]. It is recommended that a final flush with water or saline be used prior to obturation of the root canal. The removal of smear layer is still recommended as it may harbour bacteria; thus, until further scientific evidence is available, the clinical protocols should remain unchanged. Further research is necessary to be able to update the irrigation protocols for obturation with hydraulic sealers.

The concept of biomineralization has also been extended to introducing a final rinse with phosphate-buffered saline [83]. The induced biomineralization has adverse effects on the antimicrobial properties of the sealer [84]. This is more relevant in the single-cone obturation technique where the obturation is made up of high volumes of sealer.

The water-based sealers like BioRoot™ RCS are susceptible to desiccation due to the heat applied during warm vertical compaction of gutta-percha [85], although this does not compromise the quality of fill [86]. The premixed sealers are less susceptible to changes in temperature, since they have an alternative vehicle [87, 88] which includes all premixed sealers not only the ones like TotalFill® BC Sealer HiFlow™ (FKG, La Chaux-de-Fonds, Switzerland) which have been developed specifically by the manufacturer to be used in procedures employing heat.

4 Extra-radicular Use

The extra-radicular use of hydraulic materials includes the root-end surgery and surgical repair of root perforations. The hydraulic cements have been developed for this purpose. These same materials are also used for non-surgical repair of root perforations and also for apical plugs in management of non-vital immature teeth.

4.1 Chemical, Physical and Mechanical Properties

The material used for apical surgery need to be radiopaque to enable detection on patient recall, exhibit low solubility and should be easy to han-

dle. Material strength and setting time are less important. The TotalFill® BC RRM™ (FKG, La Chaux-de-Fonds, Switzerland) has been developed specifically as root repair materials, and they are supplied in various consistencies for ease of handling. These materials also show sufficient radiopacity [89].

The solubility and washout are main concerns as there are no standard methods to test the solubility and washout of root-end filling materials. The ISO 6976 [59] is not suitable for hydraulic materials and less so for root-end fillers. The hydraulic-type materials are all dosed or premixed, and this is beneficial as the liquid/powder ratio cannot be altered.

4.2 Biological Characteristics

The hydraulic root repair materials such as TotalFill® BC RRM™ exhibited good cell viabilities comparable to MTA [90–94] except at the early ages, where the TotalFill® BC RRM™ exhibited lower cell viabilities [91, 93]. Osteoblastic differentiation was evident [90]. Minimal or no inflammatory tissue response was observed in the periapical area after using either MTA or hydraulic root repair material [95]. The hydraulic root repair materials are antimicrobial against a number of strains [96, 97].

4.3 Clinical Performance and Material Interactions

The interaction of hydraulic cements in contact with blood when used as root-end filling material also shows the preferential formation of calcium carbonate [98] rather than the anticipated calcium phosphate which has always been assumed to be a sign of bioactivity. Similarly, to the behaviour of sealers, the use of sodium hypochlorite enhanced the push-out bond strength of hydraulic root repair materials [99].

Superior push-out bond strengths were observed for hydraulic root repair material compared to MTA when used in ultrasonically prepared concave retrograde cavities [100]. The use of BC RRM shows over 90% success rate used as root-end filling material [101–103] and is comparable to MTA [101, 102]. The success rates of both hydraulic root repair material and MTA were higher when scored on periapical radiographs than on cone beam tomography [102].

4.4 Conclusions

The modifications undertaken by the manufacturers to produce new generation hydraulic calcium silicate–based materials have led to the development of a range of materials that exhibit better properties to the traditional MTA. These include superior handling, enhanced physical properties and material colour stability. The materials have comparable biological properties to MTA. Further understanding of the material properties in the clinical environment is necessary to be able to use clinical protocols that enhance the material characteristics.

References

1. Lu D, Zhou S. High strength biological cement composition and using the same. Patent number: 7553362; 2006.
2. Koutroulis A, Kuehne SA, Cooper PR, Camilleri J. The role of calcium ion release on biocompatibility and antimicrobial properties of hydraulic cements. Sci Rep. 2019;9(1):19019.
3. Camilleri J, Montesin FE, Di Silvio L, Pitt Ford TR. The constitution and biocompatibility of accelerated Portland cement for endodontic use. Int Endod J. 2005;38:834–42.
4. Camilleri J. The physical properties of accelerated Portland cement for endodontic use. Int Endod J. 2008;41:151–7.
5. Camilleri J, Montesin FE, Curtis RV, Ford TR. Characterization of Portland cement for use as a dental restorative material. Dent Mater. 2006;22(6):569–75.
6. Camilleri J, Sorrentino F, Damidot D. Investigation of the hydration and bioactivity of radiopacified tricalcium silicate cement, Biodentine and MTA Angelus. Dent Mater. 2013;29(5):580–93.
7. Grech L, Mallia B, Camilleri J. Investigation of the physical properties of tricalcium silicate cement-based root-end filling materials. Dent Mater. 2013;29(2):e20–8.
8. Abdullah D, Ford TR, Papaioannou S, Nicholson J, McDonald F. An evaluation of accelerated Portland cement as a restorative material. Biomaterials. 2002;23(19):4001–10.
9. Wiltbank KB, Schwartz SA, Schindler WG. Effect of selected accelerants on the physical properties of mineral trioxide aggregate and Portland cement. J Endod. 2007;33(10):1235–8.
10. Antunes Bortoluzzi E, Juárez Broon N, Antonio Hungaro Duarte M, de Oliveira Demarchi AC, Monteiro Bramante C. The use of a setting accelerator and its effect on pH and calcium ion release of mineral trioxide aggregate and white Portland cement. J Endod. 2006;32(12):1194–7.
11. Marciano MA, Duarte MA, Camilleri J. Dental discoloration caused by bismuth oxide in MTA in the presence of sodium hypochlorite. Clin Oral Investig. 2015;19(9):2201–9.
12. Shokouhinejad N, Razmi H, Farbod M, Alikhasi M, Camilleri J. Coronal tooth discoloration induced by regenerative endodontic treatment using different scaffolds and intracanal coronal barriers: a 6-month ex vivo study. Restor Dent Endod. 2019;44(3):e25.
13. Palma PJ, Marques JA, Falacho RI, Correia E, Vinagre A, Santos JM, Ramos JC. Six-month color stability assessment of two calcium silicate-based cements used in regenerative endodontic procedures. J Funct Biomater. 2019;10(1):14.
14. Kurun Aksoy M, Tulga Oz F, Orhan K. Evaluation of calcium (Ca2+) and hydroxide (OH-) ion diffusion rates of indirect pulp capping materials. Int J Artif Organs. 2017;40(11):641–6.
15. Arias-Moliz MT, Farrugia C, Lung CYK, Wismayer PS, Camilleri J. Antimicrobial and biological activity of leachate from light curable pulp capping materials. J Dent. 2017;64:45–51.
16. Camilleri J, Laurent P, About I. Hydration of Biodentine, Theracal LC, and a prototype tricalcium silicate-based dentin replacement material after pulp capping in entire tooth cultures. J Endod. 2014;40(11):1846–54.
17. Chang SW, Lee SY, Ann HJ, Kum KY, Kim EC. Effects of calcium silicate endodontic cements on biocompatibility and mineralization-inducing potentials in human dental pulp cells. J Endod. 2014;40(8):1194–200.
18. Luo Z, Kohli MR, Yu Q, Kim S, Qu T, He WX. Biodentine™ induces human dental pulp stem cell differentiation through mitogen-activated protein kinase and calcium-/calmodulin-dependent protein kinase II pathways. J Endod. 2014;40(7):937–42.
19. Sun Y, Liu J, Luo T, Shen Y, Zou L. Effects of two fast-setting pulp-capping materials on cell viability and osteogenic differentiation in human dental pulp stem cells: an in vitro study. Arch Oral Biol. 2019;100:100–5.
20. Zanini M, Sautier JM, Berdal A, Simon S. Biodentine induces immortalized murine pulp cell differentiation into odontoblast-like cells and stimulates biomineralization. J Endod. 2012;38(9):1220–6.
21. Loison-Robert LS, Tassin M, Bonte E, Berbar T, Isaac J, Berdal A, Simon S, Fournier BPJ. In vitro

effects of two silicate-based materials, Biodentine and BioRoot RCS, on dental pulp stem cells in models of reactionary and reparative dentinogenesis. PLoS One. 2018;13(1):e0190014.

22. Wongwatanasanti N, Jantarat J, Sritanaudomchai H, Hargreaves KM. Effect of bioceramic materials on proliferation and odontoblast differentiation of human stem cells from the apical papilla. J Endod. 2018;44(8):1270–5.

23. Rodrigues EM, Gomes-Cornélio AL, Soares-Costa A, Salles LP, Velayutham M, Rossa-Junior C, Guerreiro-Tanomaru JM, Tanomaru-Filho M. An assessment of the overexpression of BMP-2 in transfected human osteoblast cells stimulated by mineral trioxide aggregate and Biodentine. Int Endod J. 2017;50(Suppl 2):e9–e18.

24. Giraud T, Jeanneau C, Rombouts C, Bakhtiar H, Laurent P, About I. Pulp capping materials modulate the balance between inflammation and regeneration. Dent Mater. 2019;35(1):24–35.

25. Katge FA, Patil DP. Comparative analysis of 2 calcium silicate–based cements (Biodentine™ and Mineral Trioxide Aggregate) as direct pulp-capping agent in young permanent molars: a split mouth study. J Endod. 2017;43(4):507–13.

26. Kim J, Song YS, Min KS, Kim SH, Koh JT, Lee BN, Chang HS, Hwang IN, Oh WM, Hwang YC. Evaluation of reparative dentin formation of ProRoot MTA, Biodentine™ and BioAggregate using micro-CT and immunohistochemistry. Restor Dent Endod. 2016;41(1):29–36.

27. Nowicka A, Wilk G, Lipski M, Kołecki J, Buczkowska-Radlińska J. Tomographic evaluation of reparative dentin formation after direct pulp capping with Ca (OH)2, MTA, Biodentine™, and dentin bonding system in human teeth. J Endod. 2015;41(8):1234–40.

28. Poggio C, Arciola CR, Beltrami R, Monaco A, Dagna A, Lombardini M, Visai L. Cytocompatibility and antibacterial properties of capping materials. Sci World J. 2014;2014:181945.

29. Özyürek T, Demiryürek EÖ. Comparison of the antimicrobial activity of direct pulp-capping materials: Mineral Trioxide Aggregate-Angelus and Biodentine. J Conserv Dent. 2016;19(6):569–72.

30. Farrugia C, Lung CYK, Schembri Wismayer P, Arias-Moliz MT, Camilleri J. The relationship of surface characteristics and antimicrobial performance of pulp capping materials. J Endod. 2018;44(7):1115–20.

31. Jardine AP, Montagner F, Quintana RM, Zaccara IM, Kopper PMP. Antimicrobial effect of bioceramic cements on multispecies microcosm biofilm: a confocal laser microscopy study. Clin Oral Investig. 2019;23(3):1367–72.

32. Meraji N, Nekoofar MH, Yazdi KA, Sharifian MR, Fakhari N, Camilleri J. Bonding to caries affected dentine. Dent Mater. 2018;34(9):e236–45.

33. European Society of Endodontology (ESE) developed by, Duncan HF, Galler KM, Tomson PL, Simon S, El-Karim I, Kundzina R, Krastl G, Dammaschke T, Fransson H, Markvart M, Zehnder M, Bjørndal L. European Society of Endodontology position statement: management of deep caries and the exposed pulp. Int Endod J. 2019;52(7):923–34.

34. Atmeh AR, Chong EZ, Richard G, Festy F, Watson TF. Dentin-cement interfacial interaction: calcium silicates and polyalkenoates. J Dent Res. 2012;91(5):454–9.

35. Hadis M, Wang J, Zhang ZJ, Di Maio A, Camilleri J. Interaction of hydraulic calcium silicate and glass ionomer cements with dentine. Materialia. 2020;9:100515.

36. Li X, Pongprueksa P, Van Landuyt K, Chen Z, Pedano M, Van Meerbeek B, De Munck J. Correlative micro-Raman/EPMA analysis of the hydraulic calcium silicate cement interface with dentin. Clin Oral Investig. 2016;20(7):1663 73.

37. Kim JR, Nosrat A, Fouad AF. Interfacial characteristics of Biodentine and MTA with dentine in simulated body fluid. J Dent. 2015;43(2):241–7.

38. Meschi N, Li X, Van Gorp G, Camilleri J, Van Meerbeek B, Lambrechts P. Bioactivity potential of Portland cement in regenerative endodontic procedures: from clinic to lab. Dent Mater. 2019;35(9):1342–50.

39. Hashem DF, Foxton R, Manoharan A, Watson TF, Banerjee A. The physical characteristics of resin composite-calcium silicate interface as part of a layered/laminate adhesive restoration. Dent Mater. 2014;30(3):343–9.

40. Camilleri J. Investigation of Biodentine as dentine replacement material. J Dent. 2013;41(7):600–10.

41. Sultana N, Nawal RR, Chaudhry S, Sivakumar M, Talwar S. Effect of acid etching on the micro-shear bond strength of resin composite-calcium silicate interface evaluated over different time intervals of bond aging. J Conserv Dent. 2018;21(2):194–7.

42. Tulumbaci F, Almaz ME, Arikan V, Mutluay MS. Shear bond strength of different restorative materials to mineral trioxide aggregate and Biodentine. J Conserv Dent. 2017;20(5):292–6.

43. Schmidt A, Schäfer E, Dammaschke T. Shear bond strength of lining materials to calcium-silicate cements at different time intervals. J Adhes Dent. 2017;19(2):129–35.

44. Çolak H, Tokay U, Uzgur R, Uzgur Z, Ercan E, Hamidi MM. The effect of different adhesives and setting times on bond strength between Biodentine and composite. J Appl Biomater Funct Mater. 2016;14(2):e217–22.

45. Deepa VL, Dhamaraju B, Bollu IP, Balaji TS. Shear bond strength evaluation of resin composite bonded to three different liners: TheraCal LC, Biodentine, and resin-modified glass ionomer cement using universal adhesive: an in vitro study. J Conserv Dent. 2016;19(2):166–70.

46. Cengiz E, Ulusoy N. Microshear bond strength of tri-calcium silicate-based cements to different restorative materials. J Adhes Dent. 2016;18(3):231–7.

47. Altunsoy M, Tanrıver M, Ok E, Kucukyilmaz E. Shear bond strength of a self-adhering flowable composite and a flowable base composite to mineral trioxide aggregate, calcium-enriched mixture cement, and Biodentine. J Endod. 2015;41(10):1691–5.

48. Meraji N, Camilleri J. Bonding over dentin replacement materials. J Endod. 2017;43(8):1343–9.

49. Shafiei F, Doozandeh M, Gharibpour F, Adl A. Effect of reducing acid-etching duration time on compressive strength and bonding of a universal adhesive to calcium silicate cements. Int Endod J. 2019;52(4):530–9.

50. Nekoofar MH, Motevasselian F, Mirzaei M, Yassini E, Pouyanfar H, Dummer PM. The micro-shear bond strength of various resinous restorative materials to aged biodentine. Iran Endod J. 2018;13(3):356–61.

51. Palma PJ, Marques JA, Falacho RI, Vinagre A, Santos JM, Ramos JC. Does delayed restoration improve shear bond strength of different restorative protocols to calcium silicate-based cements? Materials (Basel). 2018;11(11):2216.

52. Bakhtiar H, Nekoofar MH, Aminishakib P, Abedi F, Naghi Moosavi F, Esnaashari E, Azizi A, Esmailian S, Ellini MR, Mesgarzadeh V, Sezavar M, About I. Human pulp responses to partial pulpotomy treatment with TheraCal as compared with Biodentine and ProRoot MTA: a clinical trial. J Endod. 2017;43(11):1786–91.

53. Mahmoud SH, El-Negoly SA, Zaen El-Din AM, El-Zekrid MH, Grawish LM, Grawish HM, Grawish ME. Biodentine versus mineral trioxide aggregate as a direct pulp capping material for human mature permanent teeth - a systematic review. J Conserv Dent. 2018;21(5):466–73.

54. Hashem D, Mannocci F, Patel S, Manoharan A, Brown JE, Watson TF, Banerjee A. Clinical and radiographic assessment of the efficacy of calcium silicate indirect pulp capping: a randomized controlled clinical trial. J Dent Res. 2015;94(4):562–8.

55. Hashem D, Mannocci F, Patel S, Manoharan A, Watson TF, Banerjee A. Evaluation of the efficacy of calcium silicate vs. glass ionomer cement indirect pulp capping and restoration assessment criteria: a randomised controlled clinical trial–2-year results. Clin Oral Investig. 2019;23(4):1931–9.

56. Taha NA, Khazali MA. Partial pulpotomy in mature permanent teeth with clinical signs indicative of irreversible pulpitis: a randomized clinical trial. J Endod. 2017;43(9):1417–21.

57. Taha NA, Abdulkhader SZ. Full pulpotomy with biodentine in symptomatic young permanent teeth with carious exposure. J Endod. 2018;44(6):932–7.

58. Xuereb M, Vella P, Damidot D, Sammut CV, Camilleri J. In situ assessment of the setting of tricalcium silicate-based sealers using a dentin pressure model. J Endod. 2015;41(1):111–24.

59. International Standards Organization. ISO 6876.

60. Kebudi Benezra M, Schembri Wismayer P, Camilleri J. Influence of environment on testing of hydraulic sealers. Sci Rep. 2017;7:17927.

61. Elyassi Y, Moinzadeh AT, Kleverlaan CJ. Characterization of leachates from 6 root canal sealers. J Endod. 2019;45(5):623–7.

62. Torres FFE, Zordan-Bronzel CL, Guerreiro-Tanomaru JM, Chávez-Andrade GM, Pinto JC, Tanomaru-Filho M. Effect of immersion in distilled water or phosphate-buffered saline on the solubility, volumetric change and presence of voids of new calcium silicate-based root canal sealers. Int Endod J. 2020;53:385. https://doi.org/10.1111/iej.13225.

63. Prüllage RK, Urban K, Schäfer E, Dammaschke T. Material properties of a tricalcium silicate- containing, a mineral trioxide aggregate-containing, and an epoxy resin-based root canal sealer. J Endod. 2016;42(12):1784–8.

64. Schembri-Wismayer P, Camilleri J. Why biphasic? Assessment of the effect on cell proliferation and expression. J Endod. 2017;43(5):751–9.

65. Long J, Kreft JU, Camilleri J. Antimicrobial and ultrastructural properties of root canal filling materials exposed to bacterial challenge. J Dent. 2020;93:103283.

66. Collado-González M, García-Bernal D, Oñate-Sánchez RE, Ortolani-Seltenerich PS, Lozano A, Forner L, Elena C, Rodríguez-Lozano FJ. Biocompatibility of three new calcium silicate-based endodontic sealers on human periodontal ligament stem cells. Int Endod J. 2017;50:875. https://doi.org/10.1111/iej.12703.

67. Poggio C, Riva P, Chiesa M, Colombo M, Pietrocola G. Comparative cytotoxicity evaluation of eight root canal sealers. J Clin Exp Dent. 2017;9(4):e574–8.

68. Alsubait SA, Al Ajlan R, Mitwalli H, Aburaisi N, Mahmood A, Muthurangan M, Almadhri R, Alfayez M, Anil S. Cytotoxicity of different concentrations of three root canal sealers on human mesenchymal stem cells. Biomolecules. 2018;8(3):E68. https://doi.org/10.3390/biom8030068.

69. Dimitrova-Nakov S, Uzunoglu E, Ardila-Osorio H, Baudry A, Richard G, Kellermann O, Goldberg M. In vitro bioactivity of Bioroot™ RCS, via A4 mouse pulpal stem cells. Dent Mater. 2015;31(11):1290–7.

70. Camps J, Jeanneau C, El Ayachi I, Laurent P, About I. Bioactivity of a calcium silicate-based endodontic cement (BioRoot™ RCS): interactions with human periodontal ligament cells in vitro. J Endod. 2015;41(9):1469–73.

71. López-García S, Myong-Hyun B, Lozano A, García-Bernal D, Forner L, Llena C, Guerrero-Gironés J, Murcia L, Rodríguez-Lozano FJ. Cytocompatibility, bioactivity potential, and ion release of three pre-mixed calcium silicate-based sealers. Clin Oral Investig. 2020;24:1749. https://doi.org/10.1007/s00784-019-03036-2.

72. Zhou HM, Du TF, Shen Y, Wang ZJ, Zheng YF, Haapasalo M. In vitro cytotoxicity of calcium silicate-containing endodontic sealers. J Endod. 2015;41(1):56–61.

73. Giacomino CM, Wealleans JA, Kuhn N, Diogenes A. Comparative biocompatibility and osteogenic

potential of two bioceramic sealers. J Endod. 2019;45(1):51–6.

74. Lee BN, Hong JU, Kim SM, Jang JH, Chang HS, Hwang YC, Hwang IN, Oh WM. Anti-inflammatory and osteogenic effects of calcium silicate-based root canal sealers. J Endod. 2019;45(1):73–8.

75. Wang Z, Shen Y, Haapasalo M. Dentin extends the antibacterial effect of endodontic sealers against Enterococcus faecalis biofilms. J Endod. 2014;40(4):505–8.

76. Bukhari S, Karabucak B. The antimicrobial effect of bioceramic sealer on an 8-week matured enterococcus faecalis biofilm attached to root canal dentinal surface. J Endod. 2019;45(8):1047–52.

77. Kapralos V, Koutroulis A, Ørstavik D, Sunde P, Rukke HV. Antibacterial activity of endodontic sealers against planktonic bacteria and bacteria in biofilms. J Endod. 2018;44(1):149–54.

78. Du T, Wang Z, Shen Y, Ma J, Cao Y, Haapasalo M. Combined antibacterial effect of sodium hypochlorite and root canal sealers against enterococcus faecalis biofilms in dentin canals. J Endod. 2015;41(8):1294–8.

79. Viapiana R, Moinzadeh AT, Camilleri L, Wesselink PR, Tanomaru Filho M, Camilleri J. Porosity and sealing ability of root fillings with gutta-percha and BioRoot RCS or AH Plus sealers. Evaluation by three ex vivo methods. Int Endod J. 2016;49(8):774–82.

80. Kebudi Benezra M, Schembri Wismayer P, Camilleri J. Interfacial characteristics and cyto-compatibility of hydraulic sealer cements. J Endod. 2018;44(6):1007–17.

81. Harik R, Salameh Z, Habchi R, Camilleri J. The effect of irrigation with EDTA on calcium-based root canal sealers: a SEM-EDS and XRD study. J Leban Dent Assoc. 2016;49:12–23.

82. Donnermeyer D, Vahdat-Pajouh N, Schäfer E, Dammaschke T. Influence of the final irrigation solution on the push-out bond strength of calcium silicate-based, epoxy resin-based and silicone-based endodontic sealers. Odontology. 2019;107(2): 231–6.

83. Reyes-Carmona JF, Felippe MS, Felippe WT. The biomineralization ability of mineral trioxide aggregate and Portland cement on dentin enhances the push-out strength. J Endod. 2010;36(2):286–91.

84. Arias-Moliz MT, Camilleri J. The effect of the final irrigant on the antimicrobial activity of root canal sealers. J Dent. 2016;52:30–6.

85. Camilleri J. Sealers and warm gutta-percha obturation techniques. J Endod. 2015;41(1):72–8.

86. Heran J, Khalid S, Albaaj F, Tomson PL, Camilleri J. The single cone obturation technique with a modified warm filler. J Dent. 2019;89:103181.

87. Atmeh AR, Hadis M, Camilleri J. Real-time chemical analysis of root filling materials with heating: guidelines for safe temperature levels. Int Endod J. 2020;53:698. https://doi.org/10.1111/iej.13269.

88. Chen B, Haapasalo M, Mobuchon C, Li X, Ma J, Shen Y. Cytotoxicity and the effect of temperature on physical properties and chemical composition of a new calcium silicate-based root canal sealer. J Endod. 2020;46(4):531–8.

89. Zamparini F, Siboni F, Prati C, Taddei P, Gandolfi MG. Properties of calcium silicate-monobasic calcium phosphate materials for endodontics containing tantalum pentoxide and zirconium oxide. Clin Oral Investig. 2019;23(1):445–57.

90. Lee GW, Yoon JH, Jang JH, Chang HS, Hwang YC, Hwang IN, Oh WM, Lee BN. Effects of newly-developed retrograde filling material on osteoblastic differentiation in vitro. Dent Mater J. 2019;38(4):528–33.

91. Ma J, Shen Y, Stojicic S, Haapasalo M. Biocompatibility of two novel root repair materials. J Endod. 2011;37(6):793–8.

92. Damas BA, Wheater MA, Bringas JS, Hoen MM. Cytotoxicity comparison of mineral trioxide aggregates and EndoSequence bioceramic root repair materials. J Endod. 2011;37(3):372–5.

93. Coaguila-Llerena H, Vaisberg A, Velásquez-Huamán Z. In vitro cytotoxicity evaluation of three root-end filling materials in human periodontal ligament fibroblasts. Braz Dent J. 2016;27(2):187–91.

94. Edrees HY, Abu Zeid STH, Atta HM, AlQriqri MA. Induction of osteogenic differentiation of mesenchymal stem cells by bioceramic root repair material. Materials (Basel). 2019;12(14):E2311.

95. Chen I, Karabucak B, Wang C, Wang HG, Koyama E, Kohli MR, Nah HD, Kim S. Healing after root-end microsurgery by using mineral trioxide aggregate and a new calcium silicate-based bioceramic material as root-end filling materials in dogs. J Endod. 2015;41(3):389–99.

96. Damlar I, Ozcan E, Yula E, Yalcin M, Celik S. Antimicrobial effects of several calcium silicate-based root-end filling materials. Dent Mater J. 2014;33(4):453–7.

97. Lovato KF, Sedgley CM. Antibacterial activity of endosequence root repair material and proroot MTA against clinical isolates of Enterococcus faecalis. J Endod. 2011;37(11):1542–6.

98. Moinzadeh AT, Aznar Portoles C, Schembri Wismayer P, Camilleri J. Bioactivity potential of endosequence BC RRM putty. J Endod. 2016;42(4):615–21.

99. Alsubait SA. Effect of sodium hypochlorite on push-out bond strength of four calcium silicate-based endodontic materials when used for repairing perforations on human dentin: an in vitro evaluation. J Contemp Dent Pract. 2017;18(4):289–94.

100. Kadić S, Baraba A, Miletić I, Ionescu A, Brambilla E, Ivanišević Malčić A, Gabrić D. Push-out bond strength of three different calcium silicate-based root-end filling materials after ultrasonic retrograde cavity preparation. Clin Oral Investig. 2018;22(3): 1559–65.

101. Zhou W, Zheng Q, Tan X, Song D, Zhang L, Huang D. Comparison of mineral trioxide aggregate and iRoot BP plus root repair material as root-end filling

materials in endodontic microsurgery: a prospective randomized controlled study. J Endod. 2017;43(1):1–6. https://doi.org/10.1016/j.joen.2016.10.010.

102. Safi C, Kohli MR, Kratchman SI, Setzer FC, Karabucak B. Outcome of endodontic microsurgery using mineral trioxide aggregate or root repair material as root-end filling material: a randomized con-trolled trial with cone-beam computed tomographic evaluation. J Endod. 2019;45(7):831–9.

103. Shinbori N, Grama AM, Patel Y, Woodmansey K, He J. Clinical outcome of endodontic micro-surgery that uses EndoSequence BC root repair material as the root-end filling material. J Endod. 2015;41(5):607–12.

Bioceramic Materials for Vital Pulp Therapy

Stéphane Simon

1 Introduction

Recent research advances demonstrating that the dentin–pulp complex is capable of repairing itself and regenerating mineralized tissue offer hope of new endodontic treatment modalities that can protect the vital pulp, induce reactionary dentinogenesis, and stimulate revascularization [1]. The dental–pulp is a complex and highly specialized connective tissue that is enclosed in a mineralized shell and that has a limited blood supply. These are only a few of the many obstacles faced by clinicians and researchers seeking to devise new therapeutic strategies for pulp regeneration.

The primary aim of pulp capping is to protect the underlying tissue from any external stress, especially bacteria. The quality of the filling and its seal are, therefore, of the utmost importance. For many years, this seal was thought to be the only determinant of the success of the procedure. In the 1990s, direct pulp caps with bonded resins adhesive were reported to yield good medium-term results [2]. However, deterioration of the material, especially the sealing junctions, had not been adequately considered. Although the results were acceptable over a period of months, destruction of the seal and subsequent infiltration of bacteria either led to acute inflammatory responses

several months after treatment or to 'low-level' pulpal necrosis [3]. These shortcomings resulted in a paradigm shift in the underlying biological concepts. Complete, biological closure of the wound comprising a long-term seal came to be seen as essential. This was initially achieved through the use of materials with bioactive properties, followed by the development of other materials with the explicit goal of inducing dentin bridge formation.

For years, calcium hydroxide has been used as a capping material, either undiluted or in combination with resins for easier manipulation [4]. The best-known product of this kind is Dycal® (Dentsply, De Trey). Although the application of this material directly to the pulp results in the formation of a mineral barrier (usually wrongly named 'dentine bridge'), this barrier is neither uniform nor bonded to the dentin wall, thus precluding the formation of a long-lasting seal [5]. Since this material tends to dissolve over time, after a few months, the clinical situation is similar to that when no capping material was used for the treatment. While calcium hydroxide has been the pulp-capping material of choice for many years, this is no longer the case.

A capping material should have a number of specific features, of which the following three are crucial [6]:

- It creates an immediate protection of the exposed pulp in order to protect it in the first

S. Simon (✉)
Private Practice Limited to Endodontics, Paris Diderot University, Rouen, France

© Springer Nature Switzerland AG 2021
S. Drukteinis, J. Camilleri (eds.), *Bioceramic Materials in Clinical Endodontics*,
https://doi.org/10.1007/978-3-030-58170-1_3

few weeks before the mineralized bridge is formed.

- It meets all non-toxicity and biocompatibility criteria.
- It has bioactive properties that trigger the biological principles involved in the formation of a mineralized barrier between the pulp being treated and the material itself.

Once the pulp has been exposed, the odontoblasts layer is usually damaged. As these cells are the only dentin-producing cells, the formation of a mineralized barrier necessitates induction of the growth of neo-odontoblasts, as the latter are the only cells that can secrete dentin. Since these highly differentiated cells are post-mitotic (and hence not renewable by mitotic cell division, as is the case for the other tissues), the healing process requires activation of regenerative mechanisms [7].

In a reparative process, progenitor cells are recruited to the wound site by chemotaxis or plithotaxis [8]. Upon coming into contact with the capping material, these cells differentiate into dentin-secreting cells and their biological functions are activated. Ideally, the biomaterial should give rise to the following three responses: chemotaxis, stimulation of differentiation, and activation of dentin synthesis. The results obtained to date with biomaterials have often been discovered by chance, once the dental device in question had become commercially available.

Dentin is a partially mineralized tissue for which the organic phase consists of a matrix of collagen I enriched with a number of non-collagen matrix proteins. These proteins are initially secreted by the odontoblasts and then fossilized during the mineralization process [9]. The multitude of matrix proteins includes a large number of growth factors, such as TGF-β, VEGF, and ADM. Any biological (carious) or therapeutic process (etching) that demineralizes dentin results in the release of these growth factors from the matrix [10]. Although most of the growth factors are eluted into the saliva, some of them are able to diffuse through the dentinal tubules and reach the dental pulp [11].

Another way to stimulate the release of growth factors from dentin is through the use of biomaterials that trigger partial but mostly controlled demineralization when it comes into contact with the dentin. The dentin matrix proteins can be released from dentin by exposure to calcium hydroxide [12], mineral trioxide aggregate [13], or any etching substance used during bonding [14]. Dentin matrix proteins boost chemotaxis, angiogenesis, and the differentiation of progenitor cells into dentinogenic cells [15]. Nevertheless, there are currently no viable therapeutic solutions available to exploit the properties of these proteins.

Odontoblasts are best known for their role in the production of dentin, both in terms of its secretion and its mineralization during primary and secondary dentinogenesis [16]. When a carious lesion occurs, dormant odontoblasts and the 'quiescent' phase of synthesis can be reactivated to synthesize tertiary dentin known as reactionary dentin [17]. Although secretion is the most described activity of odontoblasts, these cells have two other specific roles: firstly, in immunocompetence in relation with the toll-like receptors (TLRs) on their membranes that transform the binding of bacterial toxins into a cellular signal that is communicated to the underlying connective tissue [18]; and secondly, mechanosensation due to the presence of cilia on the surface of the membrane [19]. By means of these two abilities, odontoblasts act as a protective barrier for the pulp by fending off aggressors and by the production of a suitable intelligible signal for resident immune cells residing. Odontoblasts can transform information that they receive into transmissible information that can be interpreted by the underlying tissue. Odontoblasts are also particularly sensitive to growth factors and biostimulators. When dental tissue is demineralized due to caries, dentin matrix proteins are released, and they can circulate freely in the dentinal tubules [15].

2 Pulp Inflammation and Healing

Inflammation has a strong negative connotation in dentistry. Pulpitis is usually associated with pain (which is not necessary the case) and adverse effects that lead to destroyed and necrotic pulp tissue. Treating this pain requires surgical removal of the inflamed tissue, which is often quite an invasive process and it can be difficult to determine the extent of the lesion in accordance with minimally invasive treatments. Due to the difficulties delineating the extent of the disease, the majority of cases ultimately result in a complete pulpectomy and root canal treatment.

However, despite the adverse effects of inflammation, it also has positive effects. Inflammation marks the first step of tissue healing. Inflammation helps by, on the one hand, cleaning and disinfecting the wound to be healed and, on the other hand, by triggering the secretion of a variety of substances (cytokines) that help in the healing and regeneration process [20].

In a clinical setting, pulpal inflammation is commonly referred to as being either 'reversible' or 'irreversible'. The process of inflammation either present or not and if it is, it cannot be reversed. Reversibility is considered to mean that the process is controlled well enough that it can be halted and then guided to aid in healing. When the inflammation is too advanced to be controlled, the inflammation process is said to be 'irreversible'. This term refers to a specific clinical situation associated with relatively basic diagnostic elements (the type of pain, persistence, etc.) that are poorly related to the right histo-physio-pathological status of the pulp tissue. This lack of correlation has been demonstrated for years [21] and has been confirmed with a number of experimentation multiple times [22]. Some studies have investigated markers of pulp inflammation and their potential use in diagnosis or treatment [23]. Although these markers are known to exist, more specific information remains elusive and more robust studies are needed if there are going to be reliable diagnostic tools and reproducible use cases.

Presently, without more biological information, practitioners must deal with what is currently available: information to define the patient's pain, as well as heat and electrical tests, for which the reliability is still suboptimal. More options based on observation, including controlling haemostasis at the time of pulp exposure

and/or partial pulpotomy, can be used as clinical markers. Inflammation is associated with hyper-vascularization, which can be identified by the intensity of bleeding. Nevertheless, a similar intensity of bleeding may arise when the vascular connective tissue is cut. To visualize the difference, the pulp stump can be packed with a damp cotton pellet placed directly on the tissue, with pressure applied for 1–2 min. This is enough time to achieve haemostasis under physiological conditions. If the bleeding persists, it can be assumed that some of the pulp tissue is in fact inflamed and partial removal is necessary until healthy tissue is exposed.

As there can be considerable differences from one situation to another one, and due to the variability of interpretation from one practitioner to another one, these markers are not reliable enough to infer whether the pulp tissue is inflamed or not. Thus, it is obvious that the means for identifying and testing the presence of inflamed tissue in exposed pulp are both arbitrary and inadequate. Despite the binary classification (reversible versus irreversible), histological assessment confirms that it is not easy to differentiate one from the other.

Additional research is, therefore, necessary to identify more specific markers (biological or clinical), to develop suitable accurate diagnostic tools and to improve long-term outcomes. This is an important point to consider because being able to control inflammation remains a key factor for successful pulp capping therapies.

3 Pulp Capping and Biomaterials

Mineral trioxide aggregate (MTA) gradually became the material of choice over time as the scientific evidence of its clinical success increased [3]. Sold as a powder to be mixed with water, the substance is placed onto a glass tray and applied directly to the pulp using a dedicated instrument, such as the Micro-Apical Placement (MAP) System® (PDSA, Vevey, Switzerland). The material is not packed in, but instead is placed in direct contact with the pulp and then lightly tapped into the dentin wall using a piece of thick paper or a cotton pellet. It is currently recommended that the way it is used for this specific circumstance is amended and that the tooth is restored immediately with bonded composite resin. Since it takes more than 4 h for the material to set, a host of precautions need to be taken because spraying water to rinse the cavity, for example could wash out the material that had just been applied. If the restoration protocol includes spraying dental tissue with water, we recommend completing this step first before application of the MTA.

The superiority of the biological properties with this material has been shown by in vitro and in vivo studies, as well as in clinical trials comparing it to the calcium hydroxide [24]. The dentin bridges formed using this material have been shown to have a better histological quality compared to those formed with calcium hydroxide (3).

One of the main drawbacks of this material is the difficulty manipulating it and the risk of inducing dyschromia of the tooth due to the presence of bismuth oxide, which is typically added to the material to improve its radiopacity. Multiple manufacturers have spent years developing a number of similar materials (hydraulic cements) with the aim to bypass this limitation, thereby resulting in the replacement of bismuth oxide with zirconium oxide.

A hydraulic tricalcium silicate–based material (Biodentine®, Septodont, Saint-Maur-des-Fosses, France) was marketed in 2012. Initially developed as a dentine substitute for coronal fillings, it exerted effects on biological tissues that led to an extension of its indications to include pulp capping [25]. One of its notable qualities is its ability to initiate mineralization [26] and cellular differentiation [25]. These results are ample reason for optimism regarding its long-term clinical use.

In addition to their ability to protect the pulp and their biological activity (inflammation control), these capping materials also have the capacity to release dentin matrix proteins from the dentin upon contact with such a material. This has been demonstrated for calcium hydroxide [12] and MTA [13] in particular. Therefore, these substances combine a direct biological effect on the pulp with an indirect effect by causing a gradual and delayed release of growth factors, including a number of anti-inflammatory entities. It

may, therefore, at some stage become worthwhile to extend the application area of these materials to include the adjacent dentin walls where preparation of the cavity has made the dentin thinner. The material in contact with the dentin can extract matrix proteins, which can move through the dentinal tubules (which are quite large at this depth) and thus promote healing of the pulp [27]. This is an application where the use of Biodentine® may have real potential, as it could be used to fill an entire coronal cavity, which is not the case for MTA. However, the mechanical behaviour of the material still necessitates an additional procedure in which it is coated with a bonded composite that renders the restauration more aesthetically pleasing and that prevents the substitution material from dissolving.

4 Step-by-Step Procedures

4.1 Pulp Capping

The objective is to cap the pulp when it is exposed, with a dedicated material. The following step-by-step procedure can be used in most clinical situations.

1. Anaesthesia of the tooth is undertaken first, as for a restorative procedure. The use of a vasoconstrictor is an option, but its consequences for the rest of the treatment need to be considered (bleeding control step).
2. Placement of the rubber dam and disinfection.
3. Removal of the carious tissues and cleaning of the cavity with an excavator and ceramic burs while cooling with water. It is recommended to first remove most of the carious tissue before exposing the dental pulp.
4. When the cavity is very deep, the pulp is exposed.
5. Bleeding is controlled with a moist cotton pellet (using sterile water) placed in the cavity with gentle compression.
6. Removal of the cotton pellet and assessment of the bleeding. No other product should be used to stop the bleeding (ferric sulphate, laser, etc.).

Indeed, assessment of the haemorrhage is the only technique reliable enough to evaluate the inflammatory status of the pulp. If the pulp is not inflamed, the bleeding due to the wound can be stopped with gentle compression.

7. If the bleeding cannot be controlled, the exposed pulp should be removed with a sterile round bur (tungsten carbamide) with copious water to undertake a partial pulpotomy. The bleeding is then assessed as before. At this stage, it is important to keep in mind that assessment of the bleeding is necessary, although it remains a poor clinical tool. It is, however, the only one available until the new diagnostic tools will be developed. Another limiting factor is the use of a vasoconstrictor for anaesthesia. This alters the blood flow into the pulp, and the bleeding can hence be limited, thereby providing good control even when the pulp is inflamed.

8. The exposed pulp can be inflamed, but it is not infected. The dentin cavity can be disinfected with a 2% chlorhexidine solution left in the cavity for 2–3 min. Laser (Er:YAG) treatment is also an option. Sodium hypochlorite is not recommended as it alters the dentin structure, and it can interfere with the subsequent bonding process.

9. The capping material is placed directly in contact with the pulp using a dedicated device (MAP ONE; PDSA, Vevey, Switzerland), but it should not be plugged.

10. The cavity is filled with the same material if it is suitable for this purpose, such as Biodentine®. If the pulp is capped with MTA, the bonded restoration can be performed in the same session.

11. A post-operative X-ray is then taken, and the occlusion is checked.

12. The patient follow-up comprises both short- (1 month) and long- (6–12 months) term monitoring. The pulp sensitivity is checked by a cold test and a recall X-ray is also recommended.

See as an example of a pulp capping Figs. 1, 2, 3, 4, 5, and 6.

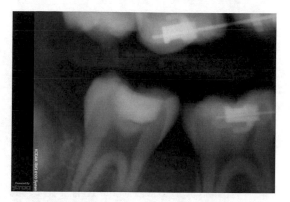

Fig. 1 Pre-operative X-ray of a 16-year-old women complaining of intermittent but acute pain. The patient was referred for root canal treatment

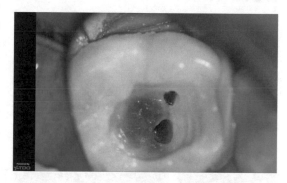

Fig. 2 After coronal restoration and carious lesion removal, two pulp horns were exposed. The buccal one was bleeding, whereas the lingual one was not. The cavity was deepened on regard to the lingual horn to remove the whole necrotic tissue and to expose vital tissue

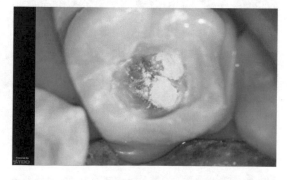

Fig. 3 Cavity was disinfected with a 2% chlorhexidine solution and pulp was capped with Mineral Trioxide Aggregate (ProRoot MTA)

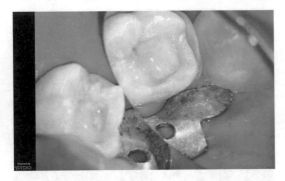

Fig. 4 The cavity was filled with a bonded composite resin in the same session. If the pulp had been capped with Biodentine®, the protocol would have been different. The cavity would have been full-filled with Biodentine® and left for 21 days. At the second visit, a new cavity would have been drilled in the material thickness and the cavity filled with bonded resin

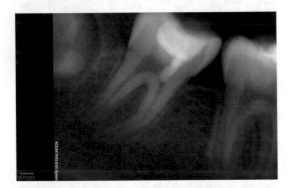

Fig. 5 The post-operative X-ray shows the deep placement of the material inside the pulp chamber

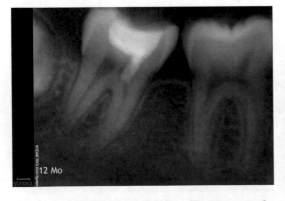

Fig. 6 Twelve Months recall X-Ray. The presence of a mineralized tissue on the close contact of MTA is clearly visible. The positive response to sensitivity tests associated to the X-ray images at 12 months postoperation leads to consider this treatment as effective with a clinical success

4.2 Pulp Chamber Pulpotomy

The clinical procedure is similar. A pulp chamber pulpotomy is indicated when the assessment of the bleeding of the pulp exposure site is not possible or in case of any doubt regarding the inflammatory status of the pulp. In such cases, it is probably safer to undertake a deep pulpotomy. The first six steps of the pulp capping remain the same, as mentioned before.

1. The pulp chamber is emptied of the entire coronal pulp with a carbamide bur used with a low-speed handpiece with copious water cooling.
2. The pulp is cut with a sharp and sterile excavator at the entrance of the root canal.
3. The bleeding is controlled by gentle pressure with a moist cotton pellet.
4. The radicular pulp stumps are capped with the capping material, as described previously.
5. The rest of the coronal cavity is then filled with the same material (Biodentine) or with a bonded composite resin.
6. A post-operative X-ray is taken to assess the quality of treatment and to check the occlusion.
7. The patient should return for short- and long-term check-ups. Note that in case of a pulp chamber pulpotomy, the sensitivity tests are not reliable.

See as a clinical example of a pulp chamber pulpotomy Figs. 7, 8, 9, 10, 11, 12, 13, and 14.

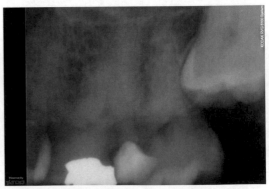

Fig. 7 Pre-operative X-ray of an upper first molar referred for a root canal treatment by his general practitioner, who placed a temporary restoration as an emergency treatment

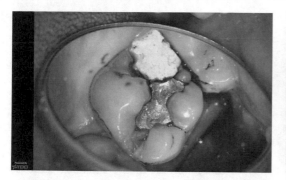

Fig. 8 Occlusal view of the crown before treatment

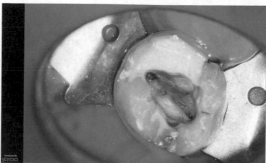

Fig. 11 A conventional access cavity was done, and the coronal pulp was removed. Haemostasis of the radicular pulp was controlled by a gentle pressure in the tissues with a sterile moist cotton pellet

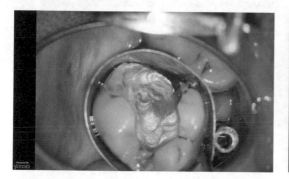

Fig. 9 The full coronal restorative material was removed

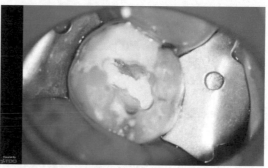

Fig. 12 Radicular pulp was capped with Mineral Trioxide Aggregate. The tooth was restored in the same session with a bonded composite resin

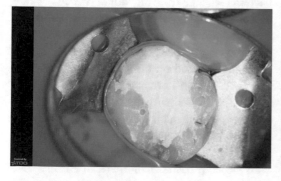

Fig. 10 The tooth is prepared exactly as for a root canal treatment. Pre-treatment restoration with a temporary restorative material (Glass Ionomer)

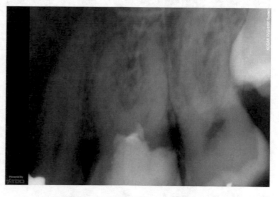

Fig. 13 Post-operative X-ray

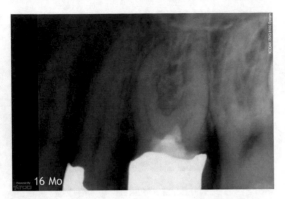

Fig. 14 The 16 months recall do not show any sign of endodontic failure. Nevertheless, the impossibility to test the pulp sensibility remains a limiting factor to conclude as a true clinical success

5 Application of Pulp Capping and 'Bioproducts' to Stimulate Regeneration

The extracellular matrix (ECM) of dentin contains a variety of molecules involved in the regulation of dentinogenesis. Attempts have been made to use ECM proteins (expressed in recombinant bacteria) to stimulate pulp regeneration [28]. The biological effects of several other ECM molecules have also been examined, including dentonin, an acidic synthetic peptide derived from matrix extracellular phosphoglycoprotein (MEPE), and A + 4 and A − 4, two splice products of the amelogenin gene. Each entity induced regeneration of superficial pulp [29].

Such biological approaches have helped to elucidate what takes place during pulp capping and regeneration. However, before they are applied clinically, more studies are needed to confirm the advantages and the safety of such bioproducts versus mineral hydraulic cements.

6 Short- and Long-Term Future Developments

Progress in the development of capping biomaterials in the past 10 years has helped restimulate interest in techniques to preserve pulp vitality. Our understanding of pulp biology continues to progress, thereby making it possible to explain the reason for certain failures because the 'Achilles heel' of these procedures remains assessment of the inflammatory state of the pulp in need of treatment. Clinically, it remains difficult to exactly know how deep down the pulp tissue needs to be removed in order to eliminate the risk of leaving any inflamed tissue. A suggestion derived from this idea was recently made in which a larger portion of the pulp is removed, thus ensuring that all of the inflamed tissue is eliminated, albeit without resulting in a complete pulpectomy of the tooth.

Until now, this treatment was restricted to primary teeth or certain immature teeth. However, in coming years, pulp chamber pulpotomies may come to be seen as an endodontic therapeutic alternative to pulpectomies and root canal treatments. In this procedure, all of the pulp chamber tissue is removed, and the radicular stumps are covered with a capping material. Preliminary studies have yielded promising results [30], although these need to be substantiated by more formal studies before this can become a generally viable procedure.

7 Conclusions

The aim of any endodontic treatment is to prevent bacterial leakage from the mouth (which contains commensal flora) to the underlying maxillary or mandibular bone, which is free of any infection and must be protected from any bacterial contamination. Based on this postulate, every clinical process that allows bacteria progression to be blocked warrants being considered.

Pulp capping and pulp chamber pulpotomy allow bacterial penetration to be prevented, merely by placing a material in direct contact with the pulp tissue. This material ensures sealing of the lesion in just a few minutes/hours and it has a double protective effect by induction of the formation of a mineralized barrier between the material and the pulp tissue. Thus, partial and full chamber pulpotomies, followed by pulp capping, should be considered to be minimally invasive endodontic treatments. Furthermore, new strategies involving coronal restoration with bonded composite resins, or bonded prosthetic restoration, now allow minimization of the indications for the root canal treatments, at least for restorative reasons.

References

1. Simon S, Smith AJ. Regenerative endodontics. Br Dent J. 2014;216:E13.
2. Cox CF, Hafez AA, Akimoto N, Otsuki M, Suzuki S, Tarim B. Biocompatibility of primer, adhesive and resin composite systems on non-exposed and exposed pulps of non-human primate teeth. Am J Dent. 1998;11 Spec No:S55–63.
3. Nair PN, Duncan HF, Pitt Ford TR, Luder HU. Histological, ultrastructural and quantitative investigations on the response of healthy human pulps to experimental capping with mineral trioxide aggregate: a randomized controlled trial. Int Endod J. 2008;41:128–50.
4. Heys DR, Cox CF, Heys RJ, Avery JK. Histological considerations of direct pulp capping agents. J Dent Res. 1981;60:1371–9.
5. Goldberg F, Massone EJ, Spielberg C. Evaluation of the dentinal bridge after pulpotomy and calcium hydroxide dressing. J Endod. 1984;10:318–20.
6. Witherspoon DE. Vital pulp therapy with new materials: new directions and treatment perspectives--permanent teeth. J Endod. 2008;34:S25–8.
7. Simon S, Cooper P, Isaac J, Berdal A. Tissue engineering and endodontics. In: Preprosthetic and maxillofacial surgery: biomaterials, bone grafting and tissue engineering. Cambridge: Woodhead Publishing Limited; 2011.
8. Hirata A, Dimitrova-Nakov S, Djole S-X, Ardila H, Baudry A, Kellermann O, et al. Plithotaxis, a collective cell migration, regulates the sliding of proliferating pulp cells located in the apical niche. Connect Tissue Res. 2014;55(Suppl 1):68–72.
9. Smith AJ, Duncan HF, Diogenes A, Simon S, Cooper PR. Exploiting the bioactive properties of the dentin-pulp complex in regenerative endodontics. J Endod. 2016;42:47–56.
10. Simon SRJ, Berdal A, Cooper PR, Lumley PJ, Tomson PL, Smith AJ. Dentin-pulp complex regeneration: from lab to clinic. Adv Dent Res. 2011;23:340–5.
11. Sloan AJ, Shelton RM, Hann AC, Moxham BJ, Smith AJ. An in vitro approach for the study of dentinogenesis by organ culture of the dentine-pulp complex from rat incisor teeth. Arch Oral Biol. 1998;43:421–30.
12. Graham L, Cooper PR, Cassidy N, Nor JE, Sloan AJ, Smith AJ. The effect of calcium hydroxide on solubilisation of bio-active dentine matrix components. Biomaterials. 2006;27:2865–73.
13. Tomson PL, Grover LM, Lumley PJ, Sloan AJ, Smith AJ, Cooper PR. Dissolution of bio-active dentine matrix components by mineral trioxide aggregate. J Dent. 2007;35:636–42.
14. Ferracane JL, Cooper PR, Smith AJ. Can interaction of materials with the dentin-pulp complex contribute to dentin regeneration? Odontology. 2010;98:2–14.
15. Liu J, Jin T, Ritchie H, Smith A, Clarkson B. In vitro differentiation and mineralization of human dental pulp cells induced by dentin extract. In Vitro Cell Dev Biol Anim. 2005;41:232.
16. Simon SR, Smith AJ, Lumley PJ, Berdal A, Smith G, Finney S, et al. Molecular characterisation of young and mature odontoblasts. Bone. 2009;45:693–703.
17. Simon S, Cooper PR, Lumley PJ, Berdal A, Tomson PL, Smith AJ. Understanding pulp biology for routine clinical practice. Endod Pract Today. 2009;3:171–84.
18. Farges JC, Keller JF, Carrouel F, Durand SH, Romeas A, Bleicher F, et al. Odontoblasts in the dental pulp immune response. J Exp Zool B Mol Dev Evol. 2009;312B:425–36.
19. Magloire H, Couble ML, Thivichon-Prince B, Maurin JC, Bleicher F. Odontoblast: a mechano-sensory cell. J Exp Zool B Mol Dev Evol. 2008;312B:416.
20. Cooper PR, Takahashi Y, Graham LW, Simon S, Imazato S, Smith AJ. Inflammation-regeneration interplay in the dentine-pulp complex. J Dent. 2010;38:687.
21. Dummer PM, Hicks R, Huws D. Clinical signs and symptoms in pulp disease. Int Endod J. 1980;13:27–35.
22. Ricucci D, Loghin S, Siqueira JF. Correlation between clinical and histologic pulp diagnoses. J Endod. 2014;40:1932–9.
23. Zanini M, Meyer E, Simon S. Pulp inflammation diagnosis from clinical to inflammatory mediators: a systematic review. J Endod. 2017;43:1033.
24. Hilton TJ, Ferracane JL, Mancl L. Comparison of CaOH with MTA for direct pulp capping: a PBRN randomized clinical trial. J Dent Res. 2013;92:16S–22S.
25. Zanini M, Sautier JM, Berdal A, Simon S. Biodentine induces immortalized murine pulp cell differentiation into odontoblast-like cells and stimulates biomineralization. J Endod. 2012;38:1220–6.
26. Laurent P, Camps J, About I. Biodentine(TM) induces TGF-β1 release from human pulp cells and early dental pulp mineralization. Int Endod J. 2012;45:439.
27. Simon SR, Smith AJ, Lumley PJ, Cooper PR, Berdal A. The pulp healing process: from generation to regeneration. Endod Top. 2012;26:41–56.
28. Rutherford RB, Spångberg L, Tucker M, Rueger D, Charette M. The time-course of the induction of reparative dentine formation in monkeys by recombinant human osteogenic protein-1. Arch Oral Biol. 1994;39:833–8.
29. Goldberg M, Six N, Chaussain C, DenBesten P, Veis A, Poliard A. Dentin extracellular matrix molecules implanted into exposed pulps generate reparative dentin: a novel strategy in regenerative dentistry. J Dent Res. 2009;88:396–9.
30. Simon S, Perard M, Zanini M, Smith AJ, Charpentier E, Djole SX, et al. Should pulp chamber pulpotomy be seen as a permanent treatment? Some preliminary thoughts. Int Endod J. 2013;46:79–87.

Bioceramic Materials in Regenerative Endodontics

Kerstin M. Galler, Matthias Widbiller, and Josette Camilleri

1 Pulp Regeneration

The field of regenerative endodontics has attracted enormous interest in recent years with rapidly increasing numbers of publications and incremental clinical impact. New biology-based and less-invasive concepts, where tissue reactions are taken into consideration, have entered the clinical routine and have changed and amplified the way of thinking in endodontics. As the body of evidence is growing, traditional treatment schemes need to be rethought. However, the idea to regenerate tissues inside the root canal dates to the 1960s, when Birger Nygaard-Østby described "the role of the blood clot in endodontic therapy" (Fig. 1) [1]. In his studies on animals and human beings, he provoked bleeding into the apical third of the root canal and obturated the coronal segment with gutta-percha and a paste made from chloropercha. He observed partial or complete replacement of the blood clot, mainly with fibrous connective tissue. These findings fell into oblivion and attempts to regenerate dental pulp were abandoned for several decades, while ambitious efforts focused on advanced techniques for disinfection, instrumentation, and obturation. New impulses came from dental traumatology, where clinical observations showed that tissue ingrowth into an empty root canal space was possible in avulsed immature teeth. This was confirmed by animal studies, where autotransplanted teeth with open apex regained a vascular network inside the root canal within weeks [2, 3]. The understanding that revascularization, i.e., the reestablishment of a vascular network within the root canal after traumatic injuries, is essential for the completion of root development was an important contribution from the field of dental traumatology. The term "revascularization" was later also applied in the first case reports on regenerative endodontic therapies. In 2001, Iwaya et al. described a regenerative endodontic treatment approach on a lower premolar with incomplete root formation, chronic apical periodontitis, and sinus tract [4]. After disinfection and intracanal medication, the practitioner detected vital tissue inside the canal and applied calcium hydroxide. Thirty months after treatment, completion of root formation was visible radiographically and the tooth responded to electric pulp testing [4]. A keystone clinical report, which sparked further interest in regenerative endodontic treatment of immature teeth, was published by Banchs and Trope in 2004 [5]. Similar to the case by Iwaya et al., the affected

K. M. Galler (✉) · M. Widbiller
Department of Conservative Dentistry and Periodontology, University Hospital Regensburg, Regensburg, Germany
e-mail: Kerstin.Galler@klinik.uni-regensburg.de

J. Camilleri
Edgbaston, University of Birmingham, Birmingham, UK
e-mail: J.Camilleri@bham.ac.uk

© Springer Nature Switzerland AG 2021
S. Drukteinis, J. Camilleri (eds.), *Bioceramic Materials in Clinical Endodontics*,
https://doi.org/10.1007/978-3-030-58170-1_4

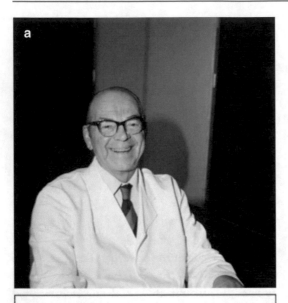

b

THE ROLE OF THE BLOOD CLOT IN ENDODONTIC
THERAPY
AN EXPERIMENTAL HISTOLOGIC STUDY
by
B. NYGAARD ÖSTBY

INTRODUCTION

In general pathology and in surgery the significance of blood
and the blood clot has been recognized (*Lorin-Epstein* 1927, *Frän-
kel* 1929, 1931, and 1932, *Carrel* 1930, and *Allgöwer* 1949). In the
healing of bone fractures the blood clot is considered an extremely important factor (*Weinmann & Sicher* 1955, and *Acker-
man* 1959). Therefore, it seems strange that in endodontic treatment bleeding is more or less looked upon as a complication to be
feared. The writer, for one, has earlier (1958) maintained that a
root filling should never be carried out if there are signs of even
a slight bleeding in the canal.

However, in an experimental study on the effect of EDTA (*Nygaard Östby* 1957) a case was observed, which suggested that this
concept needed re-evaluation.

It was decided to study how the periodontal tissue would react
if the entire pulp was removed from the main canal and the
apical part subsequently allowed to fill with blood. The aim was
primarily to see if the results would have any significance in
clinical endodontics. At the same time one might expect that an
experimental series planned in this way would reveal details of
general interest with regard to the organization of a blood clot.
When the latter has connection with live tissue at a small well
defined border only, it should offer possibilities for a histologic
study of the dynamics of the organization processes. Finally, the
purpose of the investigations was to test the effect of EDTAC on
the periapical tissues.

Fig. 1 (a) Professor Birger Nygaard-Østby (1904–1977) was one of the foremost researchers in regenerative endodontics (http://www.oslobilder.no/OMU/OB.RD5746; photographer: Rigmor Dahl Delphin; 1972). (b) The idea to regenerate dental pulp was founded on his seminal work "The role of the blood clot in endodontic therapy" from the 1960s [1]

tooth was a lower premolar with radiolucency and sinus tract. The root canal was irrigated with sodium hypochlorite (NaOCl), and intracanal dressing consisted of a triple antibiotic paste (TAP), a mixture of ciprofloxacin, metronidazole, and minocycline. After the signs of inflammation had subsided, the clinician initiated bleeding into the canal by mechanical irritation of the periapical tissues. The resulting blood clot was covered with mineral trioxide aggregate (MTA) at the level of the cemento-enamel junction. After 24 months, the bony lesion had healed, and root lengthening and thickening as well as apical closure were clearly visible radiographically [5]. Numerous case reports followed this publication, later case series, cohort studies, and randomized controlled clinical trials [6]. With recent systematic reviews and meta-analyses on regenerative endodontic procedures, the highest level of evidence has been provided [7–9]. Furthermore, substantiated recommendations from the large endodontic societies (European Society of Endodontolgy/ESE and American Association of Endodontists/AAE) on indication, case selection, procedural details, irrigants and materials as well as follow-up are available [10, 11]. The concept of regenerative endodontics is an inherent part of the endodontic treatment spectrum today.

2 Regeneration or Repair

It has been common knowledge for many years that the dental pulp possesses considerable regenerative and reparative capacity. The use of agents such as calcium hydroxide to promote healing after pulp capping procedures goes back nearly 100 years in time [12]. Thus, reports on "revascularization" of the years before 2010, which showed the completion of root formation after provocation of bleeding into the canal, raised the expectation that this procedure could result in new formation of pulp and tubular dentine and thus in full regeneration of the dentine–pulp complex. Since immature teeth contain the apical papilla, a connective tissue rich in mesenchymal stem cells, it was hypothesized that this stem cell niche facilitates apexogenesis and restoration of the physiological structure and function of the dental pulp (Fig. 2a). The presence and concentration of mesenchymal stem cells in the root canal were confirmed shortly after: mesenchymal stem cell markers were analyzed in saline before and in intracanal blood after provocation of bleeding into the canal, along with blood drawn from the arm vein [13]. Since stem cells of the apical papilla are capable of differentiating into odontoblasts, this assumption appeared reasonable (Fig. 2b) [14]. Based on histological analysis from animal studies and human teeth, it had to be acknowledged that repair, not regeneration, takes place after this procedure [15–17]. The tissues identified in the root canals were connective tissue, cementum, or bone, but lacked pulpal architecture and odontoblasts. However, after provocation of bleeding into the canal, the blood clot can serve as a scaffold and origin of healing and repair. Different cell types migrate in to re-establish, vasculature and innervation, and generation of extracellular matrix and potentially deposition of mineral lead to the development of reparative tissue, much in the same way as during any wound healing in the body [18]. As we have a more realistic evaluation of regenerative endodontic procedures today, the alternative terminology of "guided endodontic repair" has been introduced [19] or "revitalization," which is the term used by the European Society of Endodontology in their respective position statement [10].

3 Clinical Treatment

Revitalization is indicated in immature teeth with pulp necrosis, and thus an alternative treatment to the apical plug, where hydraulic calcium silicate cements (HCSCs) such as mineral trioxide aggregate (MTA) are placed at open apices. In general, a regenerative endodontic approach might be the more beneficial the earlier the stage of root development [20, 21]. From a technical perspective, both modalities require highly compliant patients, but revitalization is easier to perform compared to the apical plug. However, induction of bleeding may cause sensations, despite anesthesia. A detailed clinical protocol can be found in the guidelines of ESE and AAE [10, 11]. Whereas minor differences regarding the procedural details exist, the clinician's understanding of the treatment goal and the desired tissue responses may be more pivotal.

During the first visit, the procedure involves thorough clinical examination, field isolation, access to the root canal, and sufficient disinfection. NaOCl is the disinfectant of choice and should be used at reduced concentration (1.5–3%) to satisfy both the claim for antimi-

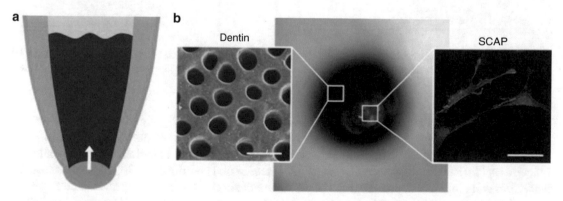

Fig. 2 (**a**) Mesenchymal stem cells are present in the apical papilla of immature teeth and can be flushed into the root canal after induction of bleeding. (**b**) The goal of regenerative endodontic procedures is to import stem cells from the apical papilla (SCAP; scale bar: 25 μm) into the root canal, which attach to the dentin walls (scale bar: 10 μm), and form a tissue that resembles the original pulp in structure and function

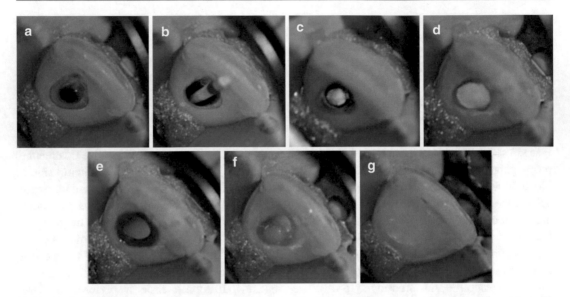

Fig. 3 Revitalization of a maxillary left incisor with pulp necrosis after dental trauma (second visit). (**a**) Removal of the medicament and irrigation with 17% EDTA followed by saline. (**b**) Drying of the root canal and induction of intracanal bleeding. (**c**) Placement of collagen onto the blood clot and (**d**) coverage with a hydraulic calcium silicate cement. (**e**) Selective etching of enamel and (**f**) conditioning of the cavity with a dental adhesive. (**g**) Adhesive restoration with a nanohybrid composite

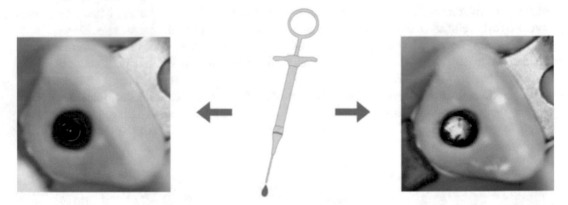

Fig. 4 In regenerative endodontic treatment, HCSCs get in contact with an instable fibrin-based coagulum full of blood cells or a collagen scaffold placed as an abutment for HCSC onto the blood clot. This situation poses special demands on the bioactive cement in both biological and mechanical terms

crobial efficacy and preservation of local stem cells and growth factors [22, 23]. Rinses with saline (NaCl) and 17% ethylenediaminetetraacetic acid (EDTA) reduce the toxicity of NaOCl to cells in the periapical region [24]. No or minimal instrumentation of the canal walls is recommended. After placement of calcium hydroxide as an intracanal dressing, a temporary seal is placed. At the second visit 2–4 weeks later (Fig. 3), the signs and symptoms of inflammation should have receded in order to progress. After field isolation, the root canal is reaccessed and rinsed with EDTA to remove the medicament and expose growth factors on the dentin surface [25, 26]. However, NaOCl is avoided to reduce adverse effects on the microenvironment as mentioned above. After a final rinse with NaCl and drying, bleeding should be induced by irritation of the periapical tissues and reach below the cementoenamel junction. While the use of a collagenous matrix is optional to facilitate the placement of additional materials, the blood clot needs to be covered with a hydraulic calcium silicate cement and the access sealed with an adhesive restoration. Follow-up is recommended after 6, 12, 18, and 24 months, after that annually for 5 years.

Similar success rates have been reported after revitalization and apical plug [7, 27]. Bony healing, the primary goal according to AAE, was achieved in more than 90% of clinical cases [8, 27].

Compared to the apical plug, revitalization offers the potential of an increase in root length and thickness [7, 27]; however, findings are variable and not predictable [28]. Failure with recurrent signs and symptoms has been reported, where insufficient disinfection is likely to be the main cause [29, 30]. The presence of residual microorganisms after revitalization may not always result in a clinical failure, but manifest in the absence of mineral apposition and thus a nonappearance of thickening of the dentinal walls [31].

4 Limitations

Previously, it was regarded as a severe limitation that revitalization procedures induce repair rather than regeneration. Today, the focus lies on healing of bony lesions and the absence of signs and symptoms of inflammation. Whereas the outcome after revitalization and apical plug is similar, more adverse effects such as discoloration, pain, or reinfection may be observed after revitalization [28]. Crown discoloration is a risk and can be induced by intracanal medicaments, irrigants, or cements used during revitalization. Especially, antibiotic mixtures containing minocycline-like TAP should be avoided as intracanal dressing because of the strong discoloration potential.

The main objective remains the avoidance of cervical root fractures at the condition of incomplete root formation [32]. Whereas apposition of mineral along the dentinal walls can strengthen the root [21, 33], the placement of a hydraulic calcium silicate onto the blood clot leaves a week spot at the fragile cervical area [34]. An adhesive seal of the access cavity and potentially at the root canal orifice may minimize the risk of fracture [35, 36].

Furthermore, long-term data on revitalization is still missing, which poses questions regarding orthodontic treatment or an alternative treatment plan for teeth with uncertain prognosis, especially before the skeletal growth phase is completed.

5 The Use of Hydraulic Calcium Silicate Cements for Revitalization

Hydraulic cements have specific properties which are not shared with other dental materials, and specifically the setting properties of hydraulic cements are improved in the presence of moisture. MTA has been the material of choice for most cases of revitalization in immature teeth after pulp necrosis and used to cover the blood clot [37]. Its property to set in a moist environment and its scientifically proven biocompatibility along with a lack of suitable alternatives motivated its use for revitalization.

MTA is Portland cement–based with bismuth oxide added to enhance the radiopacity. The main components of MTA, namely tricalcium silicate and dicalcium silicate, react with the water added and hydrate to form calcium silicate hydrate and calcium hydroxide ($Ca(OH)_2$) during the setting reaction [38]. The formation of calcium hydroxide is beneficial to the antimicrobial properties of the material since calcium ion release has been shown to be directly related to antimicrobial action [39]. The hydraulic nature of the Portland cement is well documented in the concrete industry [40]. Portland cement sets and develops its physical properties in contact with water and other fluids. Thus, Portland cement and MTA are classified as a hydraulic calcium silicate cement [41].

Regardless of its clinical success over a long number of years, MTA has several drawbacks. Besides the potential of discoloration of bismuth oxide–containing materials [42–46], other draw-backs of MTA include a long setting time of up to 3 h, difficult handling, and high cost [47]. Furthermore, during revitalization, the MTA can be displaced into the canal during its application onto the blood clot (Fig. 4). The use of a collagenous matrix between the blood clot and the MTA facilitates material retention at the desired location.

To overcome these disadvantages, optimized formulations of HCSCs have been introduced. Natural materials such as Portland cements, which are contaminated with trace elements or components that may affect the treatment outcome and success, are no longer used [47, 48]. Instead, synthetic materials are produced from pure, laboratory-grade tricalcium silicate and meet the clinical requirements. These show a similar hydration pattern as the Portland cement in MTA [49] and also generate $Ca(OH)_2$ (Fig. 5) [50, 51]. Bismuth oxide has been substituted with alternatives such as zirconium oxide or tantalum oxide, which exhibit lower radiopacity, but show a reduced risk of discoloration [52, 53]. They are inert during the setting reaction and do not leach from the material, as it has been

described for bismuth oxide [38]. The liquid component may contain accelerators such as calcium chloride along with water-soluble polymers for improved handling and enhancement of physical properties [47].

HCSC formulations are provided as a set of powder and liquid to be mixed prior to application. Additionally, light-curable preparations have been advocated due to their simplified application and quick and controlled setting. However, these are resin-based materials, where cement hydration and therefore $Ca(OH)_2$ release is limited by polymerization [54, 55]. It has also to be noted that these materials are cytotoxic due to the contained monomers, which is exacerbated by the low depth of cure caused by the filler amount [39] and thus will severely compromise their biocompatibility and counteract the purpose of hydraulic calcium silicates [56, 57]. Furthermore, the hydrophobicity and amount of filler particles will limit the passage of fluid necessary for the hydration reaction of a light-curable formulation [54, 56]. Other additives such as calcium phosphates and microsilica have been used; however, those can affect formation of $Ca(OH)_2$ [58, 59] and also compromise biocompatibility [60].

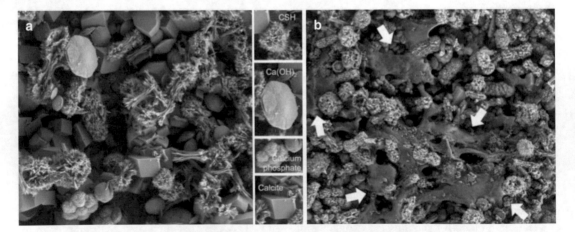

Fig. 5 (a) Scanning electron microscopic imaging of surface structure of a hydraulic calcium silicate cement (Biodentine™, Septodont, Saint-Maur-des-Fossés, France) after incubation in cell culture medium shows calcium silicate hydrate (CSH) deposits, calcite microcrystals, calcium hydroxide plates, and calcium phosphate particles [51]. (b) Adhesion and spreading of human dental pulp stem cells on the surface of tricalcium silicate demonstrates the biocompatibility of the material (arrows) [51]

6 Reaction of Hydraulic Tricalcium Silicates with Tissue Fluids

Part of the bioactivity of hydraulic calcium silicates is due to their interaction with tissue fluid and the formation of carbonated apatite on their surface [61, 62]. During the setting reaction, hydrolysis and ion exchange lead to the formation of calcium hydroxide as a by-product [47]. The alkaline pH promotes the formation of an amorphous calcium silicate hydrate gel on the surface of calcium silicate particles and calcium ions from the fluid become bound [63]. These calcium ions can be released later and react with hydrogen phosphate from phosphate-containing liquids. Amorphous calcium phosphates form near the surface and precipitate in a calcium silicate hydrate layer (Fig. 5). This calcium phosphate matures over time and forms carbonated apatite [63]. Since carbonated apatite represents the biological elements found in mineralized tissues, it plays a triggering role regarding the cytocompatibility and bioactive potential of HCSCs [51, 64]. Blood is saturated with calcium and phosphate and hydraulic calcium silicates will, thus, interact with the clot during revitalization. Whereas the bioactivity of these materials, such as hydroxyapatite formation, antibacterial activity, and induction of mineralization, has been demonstrated in vitro, it is not clear whether these properties are exerted and/or critical for the use of hydraulic calcium silicates in vivo [65]. Little information can be found in the literature regarding the biological behavior of these materials in contact with blood or resorbable collagen matrices; however, recent studies indicate that the clinical situation appears differently [61, 63, 66]. One report described chemical and micromechanical analysis of a Portland-based cement that was recovered from a patient after failed revitalization [66]. The porous material surface was enriched in calcium carbonate instead of calcium hydroxide or apatite. This observation has been made for "bioglass" before [62, 67] and further studies are required to elucidate the properties and behavior of HCSCs in a clinical environment.

7 Mechanical Properties of Hydraulic Calcium Silicates in Revitalization

Whereas HCSCs can be applied in a moist environment, local conditions and contamination can alter the setting characteristics and affect the mechanical properties of the resulting material. A compromised setting reaction and reduction of microhardness have been described in presence of serum or tissue fluids [68, 69]. Similarly, blood components can compromise the mechanical properties of HCSCs [47] and reduce compressive strength and microhardness [70, 71]. Synthetic tricalcium silicates have been found to adhere better to dentin than conventional MTA [72, 73] due to a smaller particle size and deeper penetration into the dentinal tubules. It has to be noted that endodontic irrigants and medicaments such as chlorhexidine, EDTA, or antibiotic pastes may negatively affect bond strength, whereas sodium hypochlorite or saline has no influence, and calcium hydroxide may even lead to stronger adhesion [72, 74, 75]. However, recommendations from manufacturers regarding the use of irrigants and medicaments are lacking.

Whereas in the case of an apical plug, HCSC is in contact with a vascularized connective tissue, it is a loose and fibrin-based coagulum with blood cells or a collagen scaffold in the case of revitalization (Fig. 4). Although current hydraulic tricalcium silicate formulations are adequate and currently the material of choice, it seems beneficial to design and develop more specific materials for application in regenerative endodontic procedures.

8 Discoloration

Original formulations of MTA contained bismuth oxide as a radiopacifier and induced considerable discoloration [43, 76]. As teeth treated by revitalization are frequently front teeth after dental trauma, the esthetic aspect must not be neglected. In contrast to an apical plug with HCSCs, the material is placed much further coronally during revitalization, and discoloration of the surrounding dentin is now in the visible zone and becomes problematic. The potential of HCSCs to cause discoloration depends on different factors and is therefore variable. New formulations of HCSCs replaced bismuth oxide with zirconium or tantalum oxide and thus reduced dentin staining [47, 76]. A contamination of MTA with blood leads to inclusion of blood components into the material's porous structure, which might cause discoloration [77]. Furthermore, the interaction of blood components with bismuth oxide results in dentin staining [45, 65]. As new materials are more homogenous with less pores, the risk of discoloration after contact with blood is reduced. Interestingly, formulations without bismuth oxide were also reported to stain dentine after contact with irrigants like NaOCl or chlorhexidine, however, to a much lesser extent [52, 76]. Stringent selection of the materials used, e.g., non-discoloring intracanal medicaments and hydraulic calcium silicate cements without bismuth oxide as radiopacifier, can minimize the risk of severe discoloration.

9 Conclusion

Hydraulic calcium silicates are today the materials of choice to cover the blood clot in revitalization procedures. It is important to choose materials with suitable handling properties and with the least potential for discoloration. It remains unclear whether these materials can exert their favorable properties in contact with the blood clot. Thus, further investigations and development are necessary.

References

1. Nygaard-Østby B. The role of the blood clot in endodontic therapy. An experimental histologic study. Acta Odontol Scand. 1961;19:324–53.
2. Skoglund A, Tronstad L, Wallenius K. A microangiographic study of vascular changes in replanted and autotransplanted teeth of young dogs. Oral Surg Oral Med Oral Pathol. 1978;45(1):17–28.
3. Claus I, Laureys W, Cornelissen R, Dermaut LR. Histologic analysis of pulpal revascularization of autotransplanted immature teeth after removal of the original pulp tissue. Am J Orthod Dentofac Orthop. 2004;125(1):93–9.
4. Iwaya SI, Ikawa M, Kubota M. Revascularization of an immature permanent tooth with apical periodontitis and sinus tract. Dent Traumatol. 2001;17(4):185–7.
5. Banchs F, Trope M. Revascularization of immature permanent teeth with apical periodontitis: new treatment protocol? J Endod. 2004;30(4):196–200.
6. Diogenes AR, Henry MA, Teixeira FB, Hargreaves KM. An update on clinical regenerative endodontics. Endod Top. 2013;28(1):2–23.
7. Torabinejad M, Nosrat A, Verma P, Udochukwu O. Regenerative endodontic treatment or mineral trioxide aggregate apical plug in teeth with necrotic pulps and open apices: a systematic review and meta-analysis. J Endod. 2017;43(11):1806–20.
8. Tong HJ, Rajan S, Bhujel N, Kang J, Duggal M, Nazzal H. Regenerative endodontic therapy in the management of nonvital immature permanent teeth: a systematic review-outcome evaluation and meta-analysis. J Endod. 2017;43(9):1453–64.
9. Nicoloso GF, Goldenfum GM, Pizzol TDSD, Scarparo RK, Montagner F, de Almeida Rodrigues J, et al. Pulp revascularization or apexification for the treatment of immature necrotic permanent teeth: systematic review and meta-analysis. J Clin Pediatr Dent. 2019;43(5):305–13.
10. Galler KM, Krastl G, Simon S, Van Gorp G, Meschi N, Vahedi B, et al. European Society of Endodontology position statement: revitalization procedures. Int Endod J. 2016;49(8):717–23.
11. American Association of Endodontists (AAE). Clinical considerations for a regenerative procedure.
12. Hermann BW. Calciumhydroxid als Mittel zum Behandeln und Füllen von Wurzelkanälen. Doctoral dissertation, University of Würzburg. 1920.
13. Lovelace TW, Henry MA, Hargreaves KM, Diogenes AR. Evaluation of the delivery of mesenchymal stem cells into the root canal space of necrotic immature teeth after clinical regenerative endodontic procedure. J Endod. 2011;37(2):133–8.
14. Bakopoulou A, Leyhausen G, Volk J, Tsiftsoglou A, Garefis P, Koidis P, et al. Comparative analysis of in vitro osteo/odontogenic differentiation potential of human dental pulp stem cells (DPSCs) and stem cells from the apical papilla (SCAP). Arch Oral Biol. 2011;56(7):709–21.
15. Wang X, Thibodeau B, Trope M, Lin LM, Huang GT-J. Histologic characterization of regenerated tissues in canal space after the revitalization/revascularization procedure of immature dog teeth with apical periodontitis. J Endod. 2010;36(1):56–63.
16. da Silva LAB, Nelson-Filho P, da Silva RAB, Flores DSH, Heilborn C, Johnson JD, et al. Revascularization and periapical repair after endodontic treatment using apical negative pressure irrigation versus conventional irrigation plus triantibiotic intracanal dressing in dogs'

teeth with apical periodontitis. Oral Surg Oral Med Oral Pathol Oral Radiol Endod. 2010;109(5):779–87.

17. Shimizu E, Ricucci D, Albert J, Alobaid AS, Gibbs JL, Huang GT-J, et al. Clinical, radiographic, and histological observation of a human immature permanent tooth with chronic apical abscess after revitalization treatment. J Endod. 2013;39(8):1078–83.

18. Austah O, Joon R, Fath WM, Chrepa V, Diogenes AR, EzEldeen M, et al. Comprehensive characterization of 2 immature teeth treated with regenerative endodontic procedures. J Endod. 2018;44(12):1802–11.

19. Diogenes AR, Ruparel NB, Shiloah Y, Hargreaves KM. Regenerative endodontics: a way forward. J Am Dent Assoc. 2016;147(5):372–80.

20. Kim SG, Malek M, Sigurdsson A, Lin LM, Kahler B. Regenerative endodontics: a comprehensive review. Int Endod J. 2018;51(12):1367–88.

21. Bucchi C, Marcé-Nogué J, Galler KM, Widbiller M. Biomechanical performance of an immature maxillary central incisor after revitalization: a finite element analysis. Int Endod J. 2019;52(10):1508–18.

22. Diogenes AR, Ruparel NB, Teixeira FB, Hargreaves KM. Translational science in disinfection for regenerative endodontics. J Endod. 2014;40(4 Suppl):S52–7.

23. Galler KM. Clinical procedures for revitalization: current knowledge and considerations. Int Endod J. 2016;49(10):926–36.

24. Martin DE, De Almeida JFA, Henry MA, Khaing ZZ, Schmidt CE, Teixeira FB, et al. Concentration-dependent effect of sodium hypochlorite on stem cells of apical papilla survival and differentiation. J Endod. 2014;40(1):51–5.

25. Galler KM, Widbiller M, Buchalla W, Eidt A, Hiller K-A, Hoffer PC, et al. EDTA conditioning of dentine promotes adhesion, migration and differentiation of dental pulp stem cells. Int Endod J. 2016;49(6):581–90.

26. Mohammadi Z, Dummer PMH. Properties and applications of calcium hydroxide in endodontics and dental traumatology. Int Endod J. 2011;44(8):697–730.

27. Lin J, Zeng Q, Wei X, Zhao W, Cui M, Gu J, et al. Regenerative endodontics versus apexification in immature permanent teeth with apical periodontitis: a prospective randomized controlled study. J Endod. 2017;43(11):1821–7.

28. Kahler B, Rossi-Fedele G, Chugal N, Lin LM. An evidence-based review of the efficacy of treatment approaches for immature permanent teeth with pulp necrosis. J Endod. 2017;43(7):1052–7.

29. Almutairi W, Yassen GH, Aminoshariae A, Williams KA, Mickel A. Regenerative endodontics: a systematic analysis of the failed cases. J Endod. 2019;45:567.

30. Meschi N, Hilkens P, Van Gorp G, Strijbos O, Mavridou AM, de Llano Perula MC, et al. Regenerative endodontic procedures posttrauma: immunohistologic analysis of a retrospective series of failed cases. J Endod. 2019;45(4):427–34.

31. Verma P, Nosrat A, Kim JR, Price JB, Wang P, Bair E, et al. Effect of residual bacteria on the outcome of pulp regeneration in vivo. J Dent Res. 2017;96(1):100–6.

32. Cvek M. Prognosis of luxated non-vital maxillary incisors treated with calcium hydroxide and filled with gutta-percha. A retrospective clinical study. Dent Traumatol. 1992;8(2):45–55.

33. Zhou R, Wang Y, Chen Y, Chen S, Lyu H, Cai Z, et al. Radiographic, histologic, and biomechanical evaluation of combined application of platelet-rich fibrin with blood clot in regenerative endodontics. J Endod. 2017;43(12):2034–40.

34. Ree MH, Schwartz RS. Long-term success of nonvital, immature permanent incisors treated with a mineral trioxide aggregate plug and adhesive restorations: a case series from a private endodontic practice. J Endod. 2017;43(8):1370–7.

35. Jamshidi D, Homayouni H, Moradi Majd N, Shahabi S, Arvin A, Ranjbar OB. Impact and fracture strength of simulated immature teeth treated with mineral trioxide aggregate apical plug and fiber post versus revascularization. J Endod. 2018;44(12):1878–82.

36. Belli S, Eraslan O, Eskitaşcıoğlu G. Effect of different treatment options on biomechanics of immature teeth: a finite element stress analysis study. J Endod. 2018;44(3):475–9.

37. Kontakiotis EG, Filippatos CG, Tzanetakis GN, Agrafioti A. Regenerative endodontic therapy: a data analysis of clinical protocols. J Endod. 2015;41(2):146–54.

38. Camilleri J. Characterization of hydration products of mineral trioxide aggregate. Int Endod J. 2008;41(5):408–17.

39. Koutroulis A, Kuehne SA, Cooper PR, Camilleri J. The role of calcium ion release on biocompatibility and antimicrobial properties of hydraulic cements. Sci Rep. 2019;9(1):19019–0.

40. Neville AM. Properties of concrete. Englewood cliffs, NJ: Prentice Hall; 2011, 1 p.

41. Darvell BW, Wu RCT. "MTA-"an hydraulic silicate cement: review update and setting reaction. Dent Mater. 2011;27(5):407–22.

42. Camilleri J. Color stability of white mineral trioxide aggregate in contact with hypochlorite solution. J Endod. 2014;40(3):436–40.

43. Marciano MA, Costa RM, Camilleri J, Mondelli RFL, Guimarães BM, Duarte MAH. Assessment of color stability of white mineral trioxide aggregate angelus and bismuth oxide in contact with tooth structure. J Endod. 2014;40(8):1235–40.

44. Vallés M, Mercadé M, Durán-Sindreu F, Bourdelande JL, Roig M. Color stability of white mineral trioxide aggregate. Clin Oral Investig. 2013;17(4):1155–9.

45. Guimarães BM, Tartari T, Marciano MA, Vivan RR, Mondeli RFL, Camilleri J, et al. Color stability, radiopacity, and chemical characteristics of white mineral trioxide aggregate associated with 2 different vehicles in contact with blood. J Endod. 2015;41(6):947–52.

46. Felman D, Parashos P. Coronal tooth discoloration and white mineral trioxide aggregate. J Endod. 2013;39(4):484–7.

47. Camilleri J. Mineral trioxide aggregate: present and future developments. Endod Top. 2015;32(1):31–46.

48. Duarte MAH, De Oliveira Demarchi ACC, Yamashita JC, Kuga MC, De Campos Fraga S. Arsenic release provided by MTA and Portland cement. Oral Surg Oral Med Oral Pathol Oral Radiol Endod. 2005;99(5):648–50.

49. Camilleri J. Characterization and hydration kinetics of tricalcium silicate cement for use as a dental biomaterial. Dent Mater. 2011;27(8):836–44.

50. Camilleri J, Sorrentino F, Damidot D. Investigation of the hydration and bioactivity of radiopacified tricalcium silicate cement, Biodentine and MTA Angelus. Dent Mater. 2013;29(5):580–93.

51. Widbiller M, Lindner SR, Buchalla W, Eidt A, Hiller K-A, Schmalz G, et al. Three-dimensional culture of dental pulp stem cells in direct contact to tricalcium silicate cements. Clin Oral Investig. 2016;20(2):237–46.

52. Keskin C, Demiryurek EO, Ozyurek T. Color stabilities of calcium silicate-based materials in contact with different irrigation solutions. J Endod. 2015;41(3):409–11.

53. Camilleri J. Staining potential of neo MTA Plus, MTA Plus, and Biodentine used for pulpotomy procedures. J Endod. 2015;41(7):1139–45.

54. Camilleri J. Hydration characteristics of Biodentine and TheraCal used as pulp capping materials. Dent Mater. 2014;30(7):709–15.

55. Camilleri J, Laurent P, About I. Hydration of biodentine, Theracal LC, and a prototype tricalcium silicate–based dentin replacement material after pulp capping in entire tooth cultures. J Endod. 2014;40(11):1846–54.

56. Bortoluzzi EA, Niu L-N, Palani CD, El-Awady AR, Hammond BD, Pei D-D, et al. Cytotoxicity and osteogenic potential of silicate calcium cements as potential protective materials for pulpal revascularization. Dent Mater. 2015;31(12):1510–22.

57. Collado-González M, García-Bernal D, Oñate-Sánchez RE, Ortolani-Seltenerich PS, Álvarez-Muro T, Lozano A, et al. Cytotoxicity and bioactivity of various pulpotomy materials on stem cells from human exfoliated primary teeth. Int Endod J. 2017;50(Suppl 2):e19–30.

58. Camilleri J, Sorrentino F, Damidot D. Characterization of un-hydrated and hydrated BioAggregate™ and MTA Angelus™. Clin Oral Investig. 2014;19(3):1–10.

59. Schembri-Wismayer P, Camilleri J. Why biphasic? Assessment of the effect on cell proliferation and expression. J Endod. 2017;43(5):751–9.

60. Zhou H-M, Shen Y, Zheng W, Li L, Zheng Y-F, Haapasalo M. Physical properties of 5 root canal sealers. J Endod. 2013;39(10):1281–6.

61. Bohner M, Lemaitre J. Can bioactivity be tested in vitro with SBF solution? Biomaterials. 2009;30(12):2175–9.

62. Mozafari M, Banijamali S, Baino F, Kargozar S, Hill RG. Calcium carbonate: adored and ignored in bioactivity assessment. Acta Biomater. 2019;91:35–47.

63. Niu L-N, Jiao K, Wang T-D, Zhang W, Camilleri J, Bergeron BE, et al. A review of the bioactivity of hydraulic calcium silicate cements. J Dent. 2014;42(5):517–33.

64. Okiji T, Yoshiba K. Reparative dentinogenesis induced by mineral trioxide aggregate: a review from the biological and physicochemical points of view. Int J Dent. 2009;2009(3):464280–12.

65. Schembri Wismayer P, Lung CYK, Rappa F, Cappello F, Camilleri J. Assessment of the interaction of Portland cement-based materials with blood and tissue fluids using an animal model. Sci Rep. 2016;6(1):34547–9.

66. Meschi N, Li X, Van Gorp G, Camilleri J, Van Meerbeek B, Lambrechts P. Bioactivity potential of Portland cement in regenerative endodontic procedures: from clinic to lab. Dent Mater. 2019;35(9):1342–50.

67. Hench LL. Biological applications of bioactive glasses, vol. 13. Reading: Harwood Academic Publishers; 1996, 1 p.

68. Kim Y, Kim S, Shin YS, Jung I-Y, Lee SJ. Failure of setting of mineral trioxide aggregate in the presence of fetal bovine serum and its prevention. J Endod. 2012;38(4):536–40.

69. Kang JS, Rhim EM, Huh SY, Ahn SJ, Kim DS, Kim SY, et al. The effects of humidity and serum on the surface microhardness and morphology of five retrograde filling materials. Scanning. 2012;34(4):207–14.

70. Nekoofar MH, Oloomi K, Sheykhrezae MS, Tabor R, Stone DF, Dummer PMH. An evaluation of the effect of blood and human serum on the surface microhardness and surface microstructure of mineral trioxide aggregate. Int Endod J. 2010;43(10):849–58.

71. Nekoofar MH, Stone DF, Dummer PMH. The effect of blood contamination on the compressive strength and surface microstructure of mineral trioxide aggregate. Int Endod J. 2010;43(9):782–91.

72. Guneser MB, Akbulut MB, Eldeniz AU. Effect of various endodontic irrigants on the push-out bond strength of biodentine and conventional root perforation repair materials. J Endod. 2013;39(3):380–4.

73. Nagas E, Cehreli ZC, Uyanik MO, Vallittu PK, Lassila LVJ. Effect of several intracanal medicaments on the push-out bond strength of ProRoot MTA and Biodentine. Int Endod J. 2016;49(2):184–8.

74. Hong S-T, Bae K-S, Baek S-H, Kum K-Y, Shon W-J, Lee W. Effects of root canal irrigants on the push-out strength and hydration behavior of accelerated mineral trioxide aggregate in its early setting phase. J Endod. 2010;36(12):1995–9.

75. Uyanik MO, Nagas E, Sahin C, Dagli F, Cehreli ZC. Effects of different irrigation regimens on the sealing properties of repaired furcal perforations. Oral Surg Oral Med Oral Pathol Oral Radiol Endod. 2009;107(3):e91–5.

76. Torabinejad M, Parirokh M, Dummer PMH. Mineral trioxide aggregate and other bioactive endodontic cements: an updated overview - part II: other clinical applications and complications. Int Endod J. 2018;51(3):284–317.

77. Yoldaş SE, Bani M, Atabek D, Bodur H. Comparison of the potential discoloration effect of bioaggregate, biodentine, and white mineral trioxide aggregate on bovine teeth: in vitro research. J Endod. 2016;42(12):1815–8.

Bioceramic Materials for Root Canal Obturation

Saulius Drukteinis

1 Introduction

Clinicians have used the lateral compaction and thermoplastic root canal obturation techniques all around the world with high clinical success and acceptable long-term prognosis of the root-filled teeth [1, 2]. However, these techniques require a quite long learning curve, time-consuming, and difficult to undertake [3]. Additionally, obturation of the root canal system involves maximizing the amount of gutta-percha and decreasing the thickness of sealer. Epoxy resin, calcium hydroxide, and zinc oxide eugenol–based sealers significantly shrink and resorb over time; therefore, a thin layer of sealer has always been advocated to avoid deterioration of the seal [1].

Introduction of hydraulic calcium silicate–based cements has changed the root canal obturation standards and strategies [4, 5]. The main advantages of these materials are biocompatibility, bioactivity, and high antimicrobial activity [5]. Meanwhile, due to the no shrinkage and long-term dimensional stability, these materials can be used in larger volumes without the need to increase the amount of gutta-percha in the root canal, as it is a sealer- or filler-based obturation [6]. The hydraulic calcium silicate–based sealers are recommended to be used with a single-cone

obturation technique, while the purpose of the gutta-percha cone is to increase hydraulic pressure inside the root canal and drive the sealer into isthmuses, irregularities, and dentinal tubules [6, 7]. The new obturation technique is simple to apply even for the inexperienced clinician [8].

The new materials and obturation technique have been extensively compared in vitro and in vivo studies and have shown similar or superior results in comparison to the conventional obturation materials and techniques [9–14]. Although the long-term randomized clinical trials are needed to prove the long-term efficacy of the single-cone technique, the preliminary retrospective clinical investigations demonstrated an overall success rate of 90.9% [15]. The hydrophilic nature, sealability, biocompatibility, antibacterial property, bioactivity, and ease of delivery have made hydraulic calcium silicate–based sealers promising materials to be used in conjunction with the single-cone obturation technique in modern endodontics [14, 16–18].

2 Flowable Hydraulic Calcium Silicate–Based Obturation Materials

A wide variety of flowable hydraulic calcium silicate–based materials are available on the market [19]. Majority of them are premixed pastes in the

S. Drukteinis (✉)
Institute of Dentistry, Vilnius University, Vilnius, Lithuania

syringes, while few materials are produced as liquid/powder formulations [6, 18]. However, it should be mentioned that premixed materials are not water-based in comparison to liquid/powder sealers. Therefore, there are differences in the properties, applicability, and clinical use of these flowable hydraulic calcium silicate–based materials, which can be used as sealers or biologic fillers in conjunction with a regular or bioceramic coated gutta-percha point and different obturation techniques [4, 20, 21].

2.1 iRoot°SP, EndoSequence° BC Sealer™, and TotalFill° BC Sealer™

The first premixed and ready-to-use hydraulic calcium silicate–based material was developed and introduced in 2007 by a Canadian company Innovative BioCeramix, Inc., Vancouver. The material was launched as iRoot SP injectable root canal sealer (iRoot®SP). Since 2008, this premixed sealer is available in North America from Brasseler USA as EndoSequence® BC Sealer™. Recently, this material has also been marketed in Europe as TotalFill® BC Sealer™ by FKG Dentaire, Switzerland. The materials are packaged in pre-loaded syringes and are supplied with disposable tips (Fig. 1). All three materials are the same in chemical composition (calcium silicates, zirconium oxide, calcium phosphate monobasic, and fillers), possess the same physicochemical and biological properties, handling characteristics, and are equally clinically effective [6, 12, 19].

iRoot®SP, EndoSequence® BC Sealer™, and TotalFill® BC Sealer™ are premixed, convenient, ready-to-use injectable white hydraulic cement pastes developed for permanent root canal filling and sealing applications. Indications for use include permanent obturation of the root canal following vital and necrotic pulp cases [12, 18].

These materials are widely tested and are recognized for their biological properties such as biocompatibility, bioactivity, and antibacterial activity, as well as for excellent physicochemical properties [13, 20–22]. Sealers do not shrink dur-

ing setting, but tend to expand slightly and being extremely flowable provide an excellent seal between the dentin and filling material [5, 22, 23, 26].

These materials are also distinguished by its ease of use [4, 15]. Materials are launched as a premixed and ready to use. Subsequentially, it saves time and provides a perfect consistency, reproducible between applications. They can be applied immediately and delivered directly from the syringe into the root canal using the disposable tips provided or can be used with traditional placement methods [4, 6].

Unlike the majority conventional hydrophobic sealers, the setting reaction of these hydraulic calcium silicate–based sealers is induced by the moisture present in the dentinal tubules [22, 24, 25]. Using this moisture, sealers form hydroxyapatite, to ensure optimum chemical adhesion between the dentin and the cement [21]. Studies have demonstrated that TotalFill BC Sealer has a stronger bond than other commonly used cements regardless of the moisture level inside the root canal [26]. Main advantages of these three sealers are a high pH during setting, antimicrobial activity, biocompatibility, and bioactivity when set, long-term dimensional stability [25, 27, 28]. Clinically appealing properties, such us easy manipulation and deployment, economic packaging, bond between cement–dentin, limited microorganism growth, and quite conservative canal preparation, needed for obturation.

The working time for these materials can be more than 4 h at room temperature, while the setting time is 4 h. However, in overdried root canals, the setting time can increase up to 10 h. The setting time of the sealer is highly dependent on the presence of moisture in the radicular dentin. Additionally, the body temperature increases the flowability and decreases the setting time [29]. These materials are designed and can be used with all root canal obturation techniques. It has been shown that endodontic retreatment procedures are not more difficult or complicated when these materials are used in conjunction with gutta-percha points—conventional techniques can be used for the removal of the fillings [15, 30].

2.2 EndoSequence BC Sealer HiFlow and TotalFill® BC Sealer HiFlow™

It has been shown that water-based hydraulic calcium silicate sealers cannot be used with the warm root canal obturation techniques because heat dramatically changes properties of the materials [31–33]. However, many dental practitioners have been using warm vertical compaction technique for decades and were not ready to make the transition to the simpler single-cone obturation technique [8]. Due to the recent needs, the two distinct formulations and modifications of the same premixed hydraulic calcium silicate–based sealers were introduced [34]. According to manufacturers, the new HiFlow formula of the original BC and TotalFill Sealers was designed for higher heat resistance (up to 220 °C), exhibits a lower viscosity when heated, and is more radiopaque, making it optimized for warm obturation techniques [29] (Fig. 2). However, nowadays there is no solid scientific evidence confirming superior properties and clinical advantages of the modified high viscosity sealers [29, 35]. It is not clearly confirmed that the real temperature inside root canals during the thermoplastic obturation can reach these high values [31]. Thus, the necessity of these new formulations of the original BC and TotalFill sealers is still questionable [29].

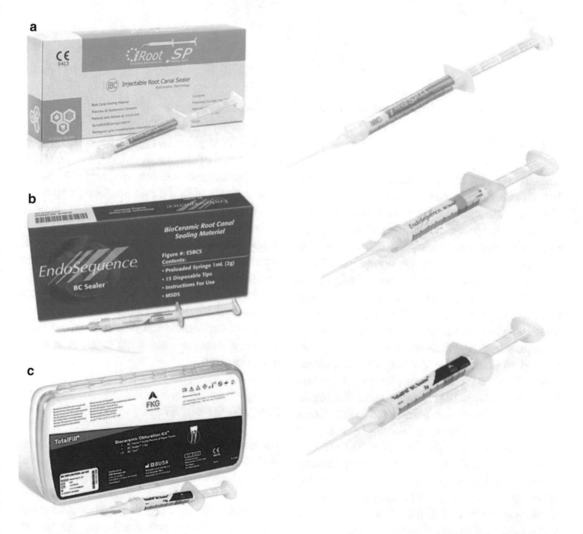

Fig. 1 Commercially available flowable hydraulic calcium silicate–based sealers: iRoot®SP (**a**), EndoSequence® BC Sealer™ (**b**), TotalFill® BC Sealer™ (**c**)

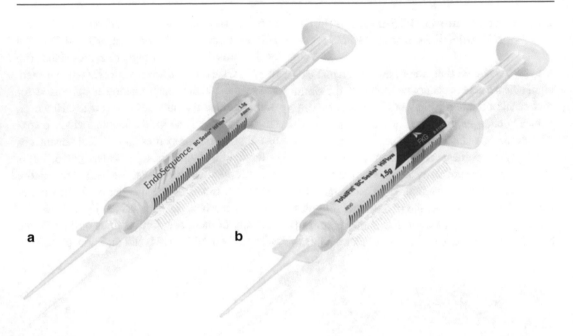

a   b

Fig. 2 BC (**a**) and TotalFill (**b**) formulations for warm root canal obturation techniques

2.3 Bio-C Sealer

The Bio-C Sealer (Angelus, Londrína, PR, Brazil) is a new, premixed, ready for use, injectable hydraulic calcium silicate–based material developed for permanent filling and sealing during root canal treatment [36]. Bio-C Sealer is available in a single syringe, composed of calcium silicates, calcium aluminate, calcium oxide, zirconium oxide, iron oxide, silicon dioxide, and dispersing agents (Fig. 3a) [21]. Overall, approximately 65% of the material is composed by bioceramic particles, while the polyethylene glycol is used to achieve the viscosity of the material and facilitate its removal and cleaning after obturation procedures [21]. According to the manufacturer, its bioactivity is attributed to the release of calcium ions that stimulate the formation of mineralized tissue [36]. However, to date, few studies have evaluated its effects on periapical tissues and related cells [36, 37]. The working time is 60 min; the average setting time is 120 min (maximum up to 240 min) after insertion into the root canal and highly depends on the moisture inside the root canal [36]. Material is highly

alkaline—pH 12.5, has high radiopacity (equivalent to 7 mm of aluminum scale), does not shrink at the setting time, and is non-soluble or absorbable. According to the manufacturer, sealer can be used with different root canal obturation techniques, including a single-cone [36]. It is strongly recommended to not overdry root canal with paper points, as the moisture from the dentin tubules is needed to initiate the material's setting reaction. Material can be removed from the root canal during endodontic retreatment using conventional gutta-percha removal techniques. It is recommended not to store the sealer in refrigerator.

2.4 Well-Root ST

Another sealer based on tricalcium silicate is Well-Root ST (Vericom, Gangwon-Do, Korea) (Fig. 3b). This sealer is a premixed, ready-to-use, injectable, bioactive root canal sealer based on tricalcium silicate, which is a hydrophilic sealer that requires water presence to set and harden [27, 38]. The material is developed for permanent

a   b   c

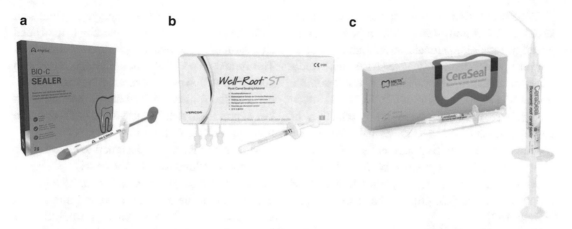

Fig. 3 The recently introduced hydraulic calcium silicate sealers–fillers: Bio-C Sealer (**a**), Well-Root ST (**b**), CeraSeal (**c**)

obturation of the root canal. The composition of Well-Root as described by the manufacturer includes zirconium oxide, calcium silicate, filler, and thickening agents [22, 38]. The material is hydrophilic and uses moisture in dentinal tubules to initiate and complete its setting reactions. The setting time is 25 min, measured according to ISO 6876:2012 (100% humidity conditions). However, in normal root canals, the setting time can be more than 2.5 h as reported by the manufacturer [38]. The Well-Root ST should be used in conjunction with gutta-percha points. It has been shown that the Well-Root ST possesses good angiogenetic properties, has a similar biological effects and low cytotoxicity as ProRoot MTA or Biodentine [39].

2.5 CeraSeal

CeraSeal (Meta Biomed Co., Cheongju, Korea) is a newly launched premixed endodontic sealer containing calcium silicates, zirconium oxide, and thickening agent. According to the manufacturer, CeraSeal is hydraulic calcium silicate–based sealer, which possesses superior sealing ability [40]. Moisture in the dentinal tubules and calcium silicate's chemical reaction produce crystallization of calcium hydroxide. The material guarantees the hermetic seal of the root canal and prevents the influx and propagation of bacteria [41]. The material is dimensionally sta-

ble, does not shrink or expand in the root canal, and prevents from root infractions or fractures by keeping its stable volume [42]. The single-cone obturation technique can be used with this material [40]. Due to the shorter setting time, the material is highly resistant to the washout [41]. CeraSeal induce a high degree of Ca^{2+} release. This product characteristically cures slowly by absorbing the ambient water inside the root canal. It is white and esthetic.

CeraSeal setting time is approximately 3.5 h, material possesses high pH of 12.73, flowability—23 mm, and radiopacity (equivalent to 8 mm of Al). The material is selling as package of 2 g premixed syringe with intra canal tips cannulas (Fig. 3c). According to manufacturer, the composition and properties of CeraSeal are very similar to iRoot®SP, while 1,3-propanediol instead of calcium phosphate monobasic and calcium hydroxide is used in CeraSeal [40].

2.6 BioRoot™ RCS

BioRoot™ RCS is the new generation of root canal sealer/filler from Septodont (Saint-Maurdes-Fosses, France) which benefits from the Active Biosilicate Technology. This unique technology allows transforming the raw material to the pure tricalcium silicate, without any presence of aluminate and calcium sulfate in the final product [13, 43].

BioRoot™ RCS is a hydraulic cement, marketed on 2015 and presented as a powder composed of tricalcium silicate, zirconium oxide, and a liquid, which is mainly water-based with additions of calcium chloride and a water-soluble polymer [25, 32]. BioRoot™ RCS has been reported to induce in vitro the production of angiogenic and osteogenic growth factors by human periodontal ligament cells [44]; moreover, it has a lower cytotoxicity than other conventional root canal sealers, may induce hard tissue deposition [45, 46], and has antimicrobial activity [47].

BioRoot™ RCS is free of monomers, highly biocompatible, and reduces the risks of adverse tissue reaction [43]. The antimicrobial properties of BioRoot™ RCS prevent bacterial growth leading to clinical failures [13, 47]. In addition, BioRoot™ RCS crystallization creates a tight seal within the dentin tubules for improved resistance to microleakage. BioRoot™ RCS is bioactive by stimulating bone physiological process and mineralization of the dentinal structure. Therefore, it creates a favorable environment for periapical healing and bioactive properties including biocompatibility, hydroxyapatite formation, mineralization of dentinal structure, alkaline pH, and sealing properties.

BioRoot™ RCS was designed to be used by manually mixing powder part (1 spoon) with the liquid part (5 drops) by simple spatulation; the working time is around 15 min and the setting time is less than 4 h in the root canal [48]. In addition, BioRoot™ RCS displayed a tight seal with the dentin and the gutta-percha (Fig. 4) and an appropriate radiopacity (5 mm of aluminum). The mixed paste is of smooth consistency with good flow which even more increases after placement in the root canal (at body temperature). It has been shown that the flow rate is 26 mm and film thickness is 45 μm [43].

BioRoot™ RCS was designed to simplify the obturation techniques of root canal, by ease of mixing and use, its optimized consistency, and elimination of the need for a warm gutta-percha technique [4]. It has been proposed that BioRoot™ RCS should only be used with cold root canal filling techniques, as the heat generated during thermoplastic obturation can negatively affect the flowability and film thickness of the material [32]. In recent times, the single-cone technique was suggested for use with hydraulic calcium silicate cements [7].

3   Bioceramic-Coated (BC) Gutta-Percha Points for Root Canal Obturation

There is still the lack of solid scientific evidence that BC gutta-percha points in conjunction with hydraulic calcium silicate–based cements ensure significantly better root canal sealing in comparison to conventional gutta-percha and hydraulic calcium silicate cements fillings [12, 49]. It has been claimed that standard gutta-percha points

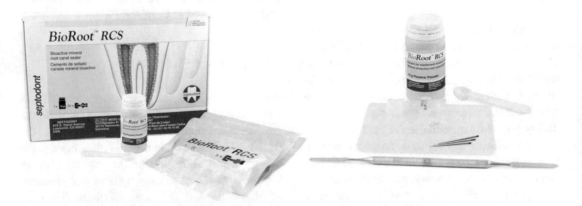

Fig. 4 BioRoot™ RCS sealer available as a powder/liquid system, requiring manual mixing before application

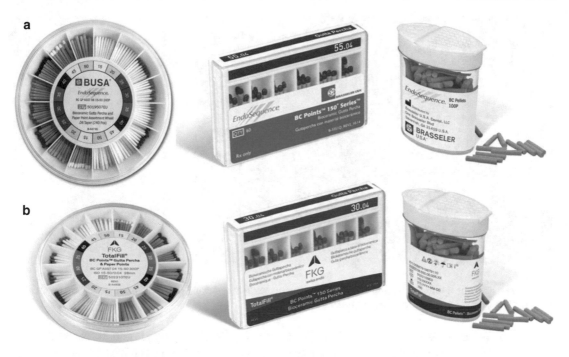

Fig. 5 EndoSequence (**a**) and TotalFill (**b**) BC points, 150 Series BC points and BC Pellets (*left to right*)

can be used with BC Sealer or TotalFill, but for a tight, gap-free seal, manufacturers recommend use BC Points [18]. BC Points are impregnated and coated with bioceramic nanoparticles to allow for bonding with BC Sealer producing the uniform monoblock inside the root canal space (Fig. 5). The benefit of using BC Sealer and BC Points is that three-dimensional bonded root canal obturation can be achieved at body temperature [12]. It has been demonstrated that combined use of TotalFill® BC Sealer™/ EndoSequence® BC Sealer™ and TotalFill BC Points/EndoSequenc BC Points can reinforce the root significantly increasing the fracture resistance after treatment [29].

It has been shown that the excessive heat can "dry out" the hydraulic calcium silicate–based sealers and thus change the properties of the materials, potentially compromising the quality of root canal obturation [31, 32]. Therefore, the manufacturer's suggested if a warm vertical compaction technique with original formulations of BC or TotalFill sealers is preferred by the clinician, it is recommended to use 150 series BC GP and Pellets. This new line of lowering melting

temperature gutta-percha points and backfilling pellets has been introduced to avoid applying excessive heat, thus making vertical compaction using BC/TotalFill sealers a clinically possible. The 150 series bioceramic nanoparticles containing gutta-percha melt at 150 °C and are compatible with most thermoplastic heat "guns" for the backfilling of the root canals. However, it should be highlighted that these manufacturers' recommendations do not have any solid scientific background. In opposite, recent investigations demonstrated that BC series sealers can be heated and used with thermoplastic gutta-percha obturation techniques, as they are not water-based materials [29, 31].

4 Sealer Delivery Methods

Flowable hydraulic calcium silicate–based sealers/fillers can be delivered to the shaped, cleaned, and dried root canals using different methods. The most popular are injecting the material, using special rotary instruments and coating the master gutta-percha point or a hand file with a sealer to

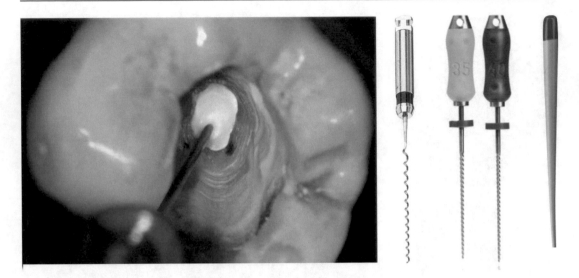

Fig. 6 The flowable hydraulic calcium silicate materials can be delivered using (*left to right*) injection via tip syringe, Lentuo spiral, endodontic instruments, or master gutta-percha point

apply it to the canal walls and space (Fig. 6). It has been concluded that the sealer placement methods can play a significant role in the sealing ability and penetrability of the sealers into dentinal tubules [48]. However, it also has been shown that the sealer placement technique is important if root canals are obturated using single-cone obturation method, but not affect the quality of obturation when lateral compaction is used [49].

Premixed sealer/fillers usually are delivered using so-called "tip delivery method," After the syringe cap removal from the material's syringe, gently attach a tip (plastic cannula) with a clockwise twist to the hub of the syringe. Plastic tips are flexible and can be easily bent to facilitate access to the root canal. According to the manufacturers, the tip of the syringe should be inserted into the canal at the level of the middle-apical third [50]. The small amount (approximately 1–2 reference markings, depending on the size of the prepared root canal) of the material should be gently and smoothly injected into the root canal by compressing the plunger of the syringe. Using a small hand file (size #15 or #20) or gutta-percha point, root canal walls are lightly coated with the sealer. After each appli-

cation, the plastic tip should be removed from the syringe with a counterclockwise twist and discarded. The outside of the syringe should be cleaned, excess paste removed. and the syringe cap tightly placed onto the syringe hub. After use, the syringe should be placed into the foil pouch and stored in a dry area at the room temperature.

If the powder/liquid formulation of the hydraulic calcium silicate–based sealer is used (for example, BioRoot™ RCS), the sealer should be mixed according to the manufacturer's instructions and inserted into the root canal using pre-fitted gutta-percha point [1]. However, the freshly mixed material also can be delivered using small plastic syringes and cannulas. After that material is inserted into the back of the single-use syringe, the plunger is reinserted into the syringe, and the plastic cannula is adjusted (Fig. 7). The sealer is injected into the root canal approximately 2 mm shorter than the determined WL gently pressing the plunger of the syringe and withdrawing the cannula until the sealer was visible at the orifice of the root canal. Such an adapted use of the small syringes for freshly mixed sealer delivery can be clinically appealing and ensure the better sealer distribution in the root canal space.

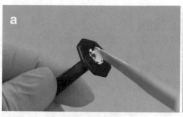
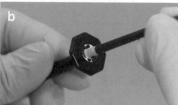
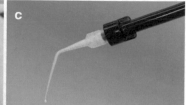

Fig. 7 Freshly mixed BioRoot™ RCS is placed into the syringe (**a**), the plunger reinserted (**b**) and flexible cannula-capillary tip is adjusted (**c**)

5 Root Canal Obturation Techniques

The flowable hydraulic calcium silicate–based cements can be used with all root canal obturation techniques. Root canals can be obturated using cold lateral compaction, warm vertical compaction, or "single-cone" techniques and their modifications [4, 19]. However, there is solid evidence that all techniques can be equally effective for root canal obturation if they are used following indications and recommendations [4, 6, 17].

5.1 Cold Lateral Compaction

Cold lateral condensation/compaction of gutta-percha is the most popular obturation method used throughout the world for many decades [1, 50, 51]. Root canal obturation procedure using hydraulic calcium silicate–based sealers in conjunction with gutta-percha points is not different from that when conventional sealers are used [4, 25].

After root canal preparation, the paper points corresponding to the last instrument used to shape the canal are selected and gently inserted into the root canal to the full working length to dry it. It should be mentioned that it is critically important to not overdry root canals when hydraulic calcium silicate cements are used for obturation, as some moisture is needed for the setting of these materials [13, 49, 52]. The root canal is dry enough but not overdried if the 3–4 mm of the tip of the paper point are wet after point removal. It indicates that there is some moisture which will be sufficient to initiate the hydration of the hydraulic calcium silicate–based sealer and setting [49, 53]. When the root canal is ready for obturation, the master gutta-percha point is selected (Fig. 8a). It should match the last instrument used to shape the canal in size/diameter and taper [54, 55]. The cone's resistance to displacement or "tug back" indicates its suitability. When proper gutta-percha point is selected, the periapical radiograph should be taken, to confirm the correct placement of the cone. Subsequently, the sealer is applied to the root canal walls and space using the preferred delivery method. The tip of the master gutta-percha point is covered with a small amount of the sealer and slowly inserted into the root canal to the final working length. The selected pre-fitted spreader is used for gutta-percha compaction. Preferably, it should be inserted along with master gutta-percha point to within 1–2 mm from working length [51] (Fig. 8b). However, in the curved root canals, the penetration depth of the spreader to within 3–4 mm from the working length is acceptable [1, 44]. Meanwhile, it has been shown that there is a direct correlation between the spreader penetration depth and the quality of the root canal obturation when conventional sealers were used for root canal filling [56, 57]. Appropriate accessory points are also selected to match the size of the spreader.

It has been recommended to use NiTi spreaders instead of stainless steel, especially in the curved root canal, as they provide increased flexibility, reduce stress, and can be inserted deeper into the root canals [58, 59]. It should be mentioned that spreader penetration depth will be significantly lower if the larger taper master

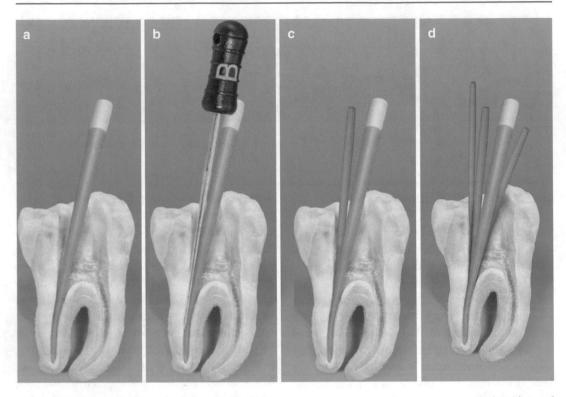

Fig. 8 (**a–d**) The clinical steps of lateral compaction technique using master and accessory gutta-percha points and finger spreader

gutta-percha point will be used for obturation [24, 60]. After placement, the spreader is removed by constant counterclockwise rotation as it is withdrawn. The accessory point is inserted in the space made by the spreader (Fig. 8c), and the procedure is repeated until the spreader is no longer going than 3–4 mm below the root canal orifice (Fig. 8d). It should be mentioned that due to the increased flowability of sealer, the space for the accessory point, created by spreader, can spontaneously be filled by the flowable sealer. It can complicate the filling procedure because the clinician is not able to see where the auxiliary point should be inserted. To avoid this clinical inconvenience, the appropriate amount of the sealer should be used. Additionally, the excess of the material can be removed by a wet cotton pellet. The excess gutta-percha is removed using the hot instrument, and the gentle vertical condensation with the plugger is recommended to complete obturation procedure. If wide root canals are being obturated, the big amount of the

accessory points can fill the access cavity, decreasing visibility and control. To facilitate obturation procedure and control, the excess gutta-percha can be removed and the lateral compaction can be continued to ensure optimal condensation and homogeneity of the filling [61]. When obturation is completed, the quality of obturation should be confirmed by radiograph, and the temporary or permanent restoration should be placed.

5.2 Warm Vertical Condensation and Its Modifications

It has been reported that the hydraulic calcium silicate–based sealers are not suitable for use with warm gutta-percha obturation techniques, as the heat negatively affects the physical properties of the sealers [31, 32, 62]. However, as it was be mentioned previously in this chapter, just water-based hydraulic calcium silicate–based sealers, such as BioRoot™ RCS, are sensitive to the heat and should be used with cold obturation techniques [52, 63]. Meanwhile, all premixed materials can be used with all cold and thermoplastic obturation techniques at the higher temperatures can be used with no restrictions [14, 29, 31]. Therefore, the clinicians have plenty of choices how to apply and use the new hydraulic calcium silicate–based sealers with thermoplastic obturation techniques.

After the canal was dried with the paper point, the master gutta-percha point is selected (Fig. 9). Preferably, it should be 0.5–2 mm shorter of the correct working length with resistance to displacement or "tug back." If the point is too loose, it can be adjusted by removing the tip in 0.5 mm increments with sterile scalpel or scissors. Afterwards, the largest heat plugger that will go to within 5 mm of the working length without binding but no closer than 3 mm should be selected and confirmed working length should be set using a rubber stopper. The sealer should be delivered into the canal using a preferable technique described above. The apical third of the master gutta-percha point is covered with a sealer, gently placed into the canal, and the coronal portion is removed with a hot instrument, while the remaining gutta-percha will be softened. The cold plugger is used to condense the softened gutta-percha and force the plasticized material apically. The procedure is repeated until the apical third of the canal has been obturated. The middle and coronal root canal thirds are backfilled, using small pieces of gutta-percha, preferably previously introduced BC gutta-percha pellets, applying heat, and condensing the softened gutta-percha with a plugger. When root canal obturation is completed, the periapical X-ray should be taken, to confirm the quality of obturation.

The recent and the most popular modification of the "classic" warm vertical compaction is the continuous wave compaction technique. The technique uses special dual wired or cordless devices combining both down-pack handpiece heat carrier and backfill handpieces using special gutta-percha cartridges (Fig. 10a). The GP cone is measured with the appropriate tip size and

taper and 0.5–2 mm shorter of the WL, while the heat plugger is pre-fitted to fit approximately 5 mm from the WL (Fig. 11). The premixed or freshly prepared hydraulic calcium silicate–based sealer is delivered into the root canal, and master gutta-percha point is inserted. Activated heat plugger is used to remove coronal excess of gutta-percha. Material compaction in the canal orifice and coronal part is initiated with a cold plugger. Subsequently, the firm pressure to the plugger is applied, the heat is activated, and plugger is rapidly moved apically into the root canal to within 5 mm of the working length. Then the heat is deactivated and continued apical pressure for approximately 5–10 s is applied. When the gutta-percha has cooled, the heat is activated for a 1 s to separate filling material and plugger and it is withdrawn. Selected small hand plugger is used for gentle compaction the remaining gutta-percha apically. At this point, apical obturation should be confirmed radiographically. The backfill procedure is performed by using a backfill handpiece and thermoplastic injection technique. The heated applicator needle is inserted into the canal, allowing the tip to heat the apical plug of gutta-percha for approximately 2–5 s. The handpiece is activated, and softened gutta-percha is extruded into the root canal.

In small and narrow canals, the gutta-percha can be delivered and obturation completed in one step. However, in larger canals, it is recommended to deliver the warm gutta-percha in 3–5 mm increments coronally until the canal orifice will be reached. The larger stainless steel hand plugger is used to compact extruded gutta-percha reducing the shrinkage that may occur during cooling. Depending on the size of the root canal, it can be obturated in 1–3 steps until the canal is completely filled. Moreover, for the backfill procedure, the special backfill guns, suitable with gutta-percha pellets instead special cartridges, can be used (Fig. 10b). Softened gutta-percha is injecting in the small increments and condensing the material as described below. The use of the BC gutta-percha pellets in conjunction with bioceramic sealers can be advantageous in comparison to regular gutta-percha

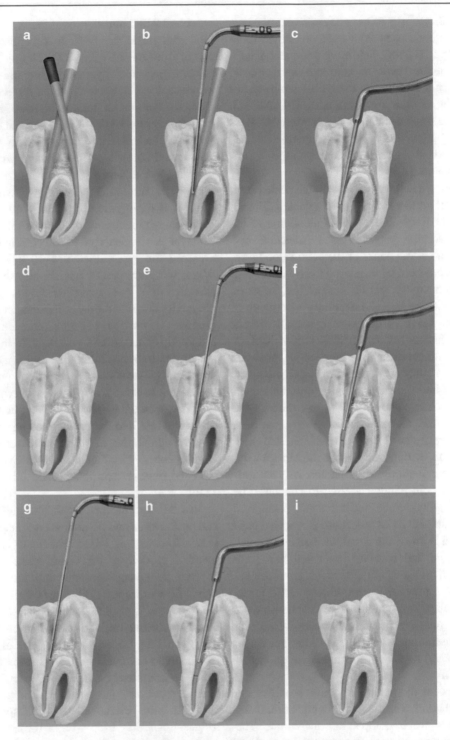

Fig. 9 The "classic" warm vertical compaction technique. A master gutta-percha point is selected and fit 0.5–2.0 mm short of the working length (**a**). Heat is applied, and coronal part of master gutta-percha point is removed using plugger (**b**). The cold plugger is used to compact the softened gutta-percha apically (**c**). Down-pack or apical compaction is completed (**d**). A gutta-percha pellet is placed in the canal, and heat is applied (**e**). The heated pellet is condensed apically with a cold plugger (**f**). The procedure is repeated in the middle and coronal thirds of the canal by delivering and heating pellets of gutta-percha (**g**). A cold plugger is used to compact the softened gutta-percha (**h**). Completely obturated root canal (**i**)

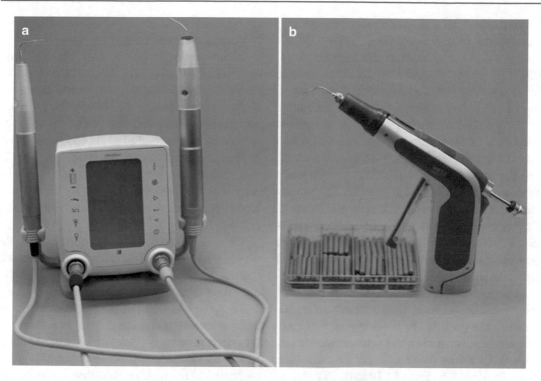

Fig. 10 Devices for continuous wave compaction technique: wired Elements™ Obturation Unit for down-pack and backfill (**a**) and cordless backfill gun-handpiece for use with gutta-percha pellets (**b**)

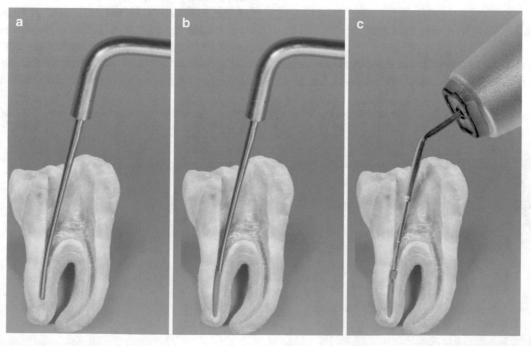

Fig. 11 The main clinical steps of the continuous wave compaction technique using Elements™ Obturation Unit: pre-fitting of the Buchanan Plugger (**a**); activation of the plugger and vertical compaction (**b**); backfill using motorized extruder (**c**)

backfills, as it should ensure more uniform root canal filling [64]. However, there is no solid scientific evidence to confirm this hypothesis [4, 65]. The quality of obturation should be verified by X-ray, endodontic access cleaned and isolated with a temporary or permanent filling material.

It should be mentioned that due to the unique properties of the highly flowable and dimensionally stable hydraulic calcium silicate–based sealers, the down-pack procedure became easier and should not be performed so precisely in comparison to cases, when conventional sealers are used. Conventional sealers shrink over the time, so precise condensation of the gutta-percha seeking to pull the sealer of root canal walls and replace it with heat softened GP was necessary, thereby thinning the sealer layer as much as possible. However, the hydraulic calcium silicate–based sealers are dimensionally stable and flows into all root canal irregularities, isthmuses, and dentinal tubules [11, 29, 49]. Therefore, the thickness of the sealer layer is not important to ensure the high-quality obturation, even if the minimal condensation to softened gutta-percha is applied [31, 64–66].

5.3 Single-Cone Obturation

The unique properties of the flowable hydraulic calcium silicate–based sealers have led to the introduction in clinical practice of simplified root canal filling technique known as a "single cone" obturation technique [12, 15]. The concept basically relies on the use the flowable hydraulic tricalcium silicate sealer–filler and single gutta-percha point, corresponding the size and the taper of the last instrument, used for the root canal preparation [4, 31]. The preliminary clinical results of using this simplified obturation technique in conjunction with hydraulic sealers have shown that it is equally effective as lateral compaction or thermoplastic obturation [12, 14, 17].

The use of cold hydraulic obturation technique with hydraulic calcium silicate–based sealers is not complicated and is clinically appealing [8, 15]. After the root canal cleaning and shaping is completed, the root canal is dried, and the master gutta-percha point is selected as described previously (Fig. 12a). It is very important to remember that root canals should not be overdried as the residual moisture is needed for setting of the hydraulic calcium silicate–based sealers [24, 25]. It is recommended to use a gutta-percha point of the same size and taper as the last endodontic instrument, used for root canal enlargement [4, 6, 67]. The sealers/fillers should be prepared according to the manufacturer's instructions and delivered to the root canal using all the conventional methods. Due to

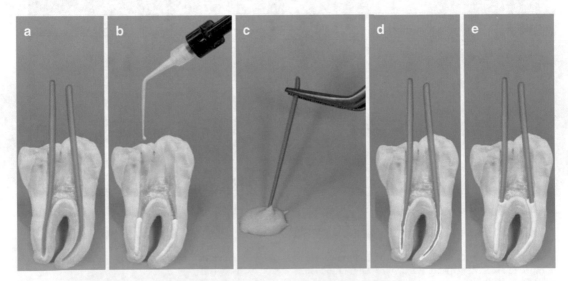

Fig. 12 (**a–e**) Main clinical steps of the single-cone obturation technique, using flowable hydraulic calcium silicate–based sealer BioRoot™ RCS and a single gutta-percha point

the high flowability of the hydraulic calcium silicate materials, the injectable delivery method can be superior because a larger amount of sealer is delivered and it is better distributed in the root canal [4, 6, 68] (Fig. 12b). If premixed sealers in syringes are used, no mixing preparation is required. When the sealer has been placed, the tip of the pre-fitted gutta-percha point is covered with the sealer (Fig. 12c), and the point is inserted into the root canal by the full WL (Fig. 12d, e).

The gutta-percha must be inserted very slowly as its rapid movement increases the possibility of the sealer being extruded into periapical tissues and the formation of the voids in the sealer/filler mass [4, 6, 69]. The master gutta-percha point generates hydraulic pressure in the root canal, resulting in a better distribution of the sealer in the root canal space, irregularities, and isthmuses

as well as facilitating material penetration into dentinal tubules [13, 31, 69]. In addition, the gutta-percha point enables to retreat the root canals filled with this technique, if the failure occurs. The master gutta-percha point should be removed by a hot instrument at the level of the root canal orifices and endo access should be cleaned with a wet cotton pellet. If the root canal is very wide, accessory gutta-percha points can be added passively along with master gutta-percha point without any condensation. However, it is not necessary as the hydraulic tricalcium silicate–based sealers are used as biological fillers which do not shrink, and it is not necessary to minimize the amount of the sealer inside the root canal [8, 17].

The single-cone obturation technique is very simple, does not require a long learning curve, and is easily managed by clinicians. The prelimi-

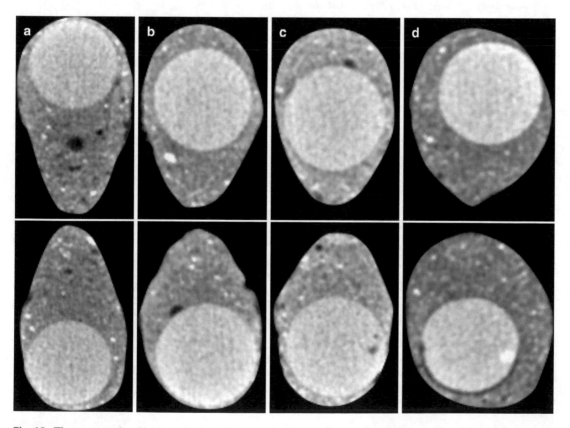

Fig. 13 The cross-sectional images of micro-CT scans of the root canals, obturated with BioRoot™ RCS and single GP point by general practitioner (**a**), endodontist (**b**), postgraduate endodontology student (**c**), and fourth-year dental student (**d**) (*unpublished data*)

nary microcomputer tomographic evaluation revealed that the quality of root canal obturation using a single gutta-percha point and hydraulic tricalcium silicate–based sealer BioRoot™ RCS was the same regardless of who performed the root canal filling: general practitioner, endodontist, postgraduate endodontology student, or fourth-year dental student (Fig. 13). This clearly demonstrates that the quality of the root canal obturation using this simplified technique is not depending on the clinical experience and manual skills of the operator.

The cold lateral compaction or warm vertical compaction techniques are much more complicated to apply clinically, are quite expensive, and time consuming [15, 51]. It has been shown that apical third of the curved canals often is filled just with a master gutta-percha point because it is complicated and unrealistic to insert spreader and accessory gutta-percha points at the desir-

able length in the curved roots [70, 71]. Although there is a lack of long-term clinical trials, confirming the clinical performance of cold hydraulic obturation technique, it has already been reported that the clinical success rate of the cold hydraulic obturation method using a single gutta-percha point and a flowable bioceramic sealer based on tricalcium silicate reaches 90.9% [15, 72]. Recently, it has been shown that retreatability of the cases, when hydraulic calcium silicate sealers in conjunction with the single gutta-percha cone technique were used is not more complicated or challenging in comparison to other obturation materials and techniques [30, 73, 74]. The simplified root canal obturation technique, when used with the stable, biocompatible, and bioactive sealers-fillers, seems promising and clinically appealing technique even in a difficult cases of endodontic retreatment (Fig. 14).

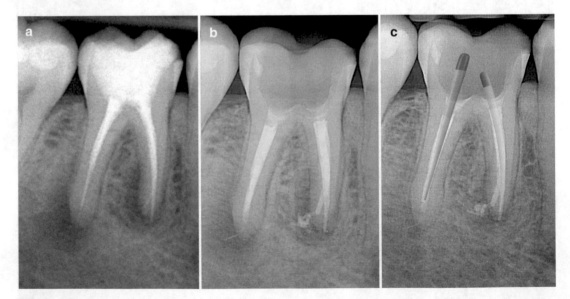

Fig. 14 Apical periodontitis of 46 (**a**–**c**) and 36 (**d**–**f**) teeth with extensive periapical lesions (**a**, **d**). Endodontic retreatment performed using conventional cleaning and shaping protocol and 1-week calcium hydroxide therapy. Root canals were obturated with BioRoot™ RCS sealer (**b**) and TotalFill BC sealer (**e**) in conjunction with a big taper single gutta-percha point. Noticeable healing of the periapical tissues 8 months after endodontic retreatment (**c**, **f**)

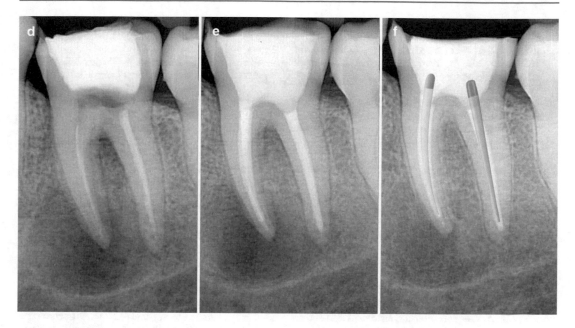

Fig. 14 (continued)

6 Conclusions

Majority of modern commercially available flowable hydraulic calcium silicate materials have particularly the same chemical composition and possess mainly the same physical, biological, and handling characteristic. Nowadays, hydraulic calcium silicate sealers are widely researched and the clinical effectiveness of the single-cone obturation technique when these materials are used is confirmed. However, the decision for the clinician to change materials and techniques is very complicated and not an easy task in everyday clinical practice. The solid scientific background indicates that the biocompatible, bioactive, and antibacterial hydraulic calcium silicate materials that slightly expand upon setting and remain dimensionally stable in conjunction with the simplified single-cone obturation can provide much better results than lateral condensation and can replace it as the most efficient endodontic sealing method.

References

1. Whitworth J. Methods of filling root canals: principles and practices. Endod Top. 2005;12:2–24.
2. Ng YL, Mann V, Rahbaran S, Lewsey J, Gulabivala K. Outcome of primary root canal treatment: systematic review of the literature - Part 2. Influence of clinical factors. Int Endod J. 2008;41:6–31.
3. Gok T, Capar ID, Akcay I, Keles A. Evaluation of different techniques for filling simulated c-shaped canals of 3-dimensional printed resin teeth. J Endod. 2017;43:1559–64.
4. Camilleri J. Will bioceramics be the future root canal filling materials? Curr Oral Heal Reports. 2017;4:228–38.
5. Al-Haddad A, Aziz ZACA. Bioceramic-based root canal sealers: a review. Int J Biomater. 2016;2016:9753210. https://doi.org/10.1155/2016/9753210.
6. Debelian G, Trope M. The use of premixed bioceramic materials in endodontics. G Ital Endod. 2016;30:70–80.
7. Jeong JW, DeGraft-Johnson A, Dorn SO, Di Fiore PM. Dentinal tubule penetration of a calcium silicate–based root canal sealer with different obturation methods. J Endod. 2017;43:633–7.
8. Guivarc'h M, Jeanneau C, Giraud T, Pommel L, About I, Azim AA, et al. An international survey on the use of calcium silicate-based sealers in non-

surgical endodontic treatment. Clin Oral Investig. 2020;24:417–24.

9. Zhou HM, Du TF, Shen Y, Wang ZJ, Zheng YF, Haapasalo M. In vitro cytotoxicity of calcium silicate-containing endodontic sealers. J Endod. 2015;41:56–61.

10. Candeiro GTM, Moura-Netto C, D'Almeida-Couto RS, Azambuja-Júnior N, Marques MM, Cai S, et al. Cytotoxicity, genotoxicity and antibacterial effectiveness of a bioceramic endodontic sealer. Int Endod J. 2016;49:858–64.

11. Candeiro GTDM, Correia FC, Duarte MAH, Ribeiro-Siqueira DC, Gavini G. Evaluation of radiopacity, pH, release of calcium ions, and flow of a bioceramic root canal sealer. J Endod. 2012;38:842–5.

12. Silva Almeida LH, Moraes RR, Morgental RD, Pappen FG. Are premixed calcium silicate–based endodontic sealers comparable to conventional materials? A systematic review of in vitro studies. J Endod. 2017;43:527–35.

13. Khalil I, Naaman A, Camilleri J. Properties of tricalcium silicate sealers. J Endod. 2016;42:1529–35.

14. Zavattini A, Knight A, Foschi F, Mannocci F. Outcome of root canal treatments using a new calcium silicate root canal sealer: a non-randomized clinical trial. J Clin Med. 2020;9:782. https://doi.org/10.3390/jcm9030782.

15. Chybowski EA, Glickman GN, Patel Y, Fleury A, Solomon E, He J. Clinical outcome of non-surgical root canal treatment using a single-cone technique with endosequence bioceramic sealer: a retrospective analysis. J Endod. 2018;44:941–5.

16. Fonseca B, Coelho MS, Bueno CEDS, Fontana CE, Martin AS, Rocha DGP. Assessment of extrusion and postoperative pain of a bioceramic and resin-based root canal sealer. Eur J Dent. 2019;13:343–8.

17. Roizenblit RN, Soares FO, Lopes RT, dos Santos BC, Gusman H. Root canal filling quality of mandibular molars with EndoSequence BC and AH Plus sealers: a micro-CT study. Aust Endod J. 2020;46:82. https://doi.org/10.1111/aej.12373.

18. Jafari F, Jafari S. Composition and physicochemical properties of calcium silicate-based sealers: a review article. J Clin Exp Dent. 2017;9:1249–55.

19. Trope M, Bunes A, Debelian G. Root filling materials and techniques: bioceramics a new hope? Endod Top. 2015;32:86–96.

20. López-García S, Pecci-Lloret MR, Guerrero-Gironés J, Pecci-Lloret MP, Lozano A, Llena C, et al. Comparative cytocompatibility and mineralization potential of Bio-C Sealer and TotalFill BC Sealer. Materials (Basel). 2019;12:3087. https://doi.org/10.3390/ma12193087.

21. Zordan-Bronzel CL, Esteves Torres FF, Tanomaru-Filho M, Chávez-Andrade GM, Bosso-Martelo R, Guerreiro-Tanomaru JM. Evaluation of physicochemical properties of a new calcium silicate–based sealer, Bio-C Sealer. J Endod. 2019;45:1248–52.

22. Yang DK, Kim S, Park JW, Kim E, Shin SJ. Different setting conditions affect surface characteristics and microhardness of calcium silicate-based sealers. Scanning. 2018;2018:7136345. https://doi.org/10.1155/2018/7136345.

23. Boyadzhieva E, Dimitrova S, Filipov I, Zagorchev P. Setting time and solubility of premixed bioceramic root canal sealer when applied with warm gutta percha obturation techniques. IOSR J Dent Med Sci. 2017;16:125–9.

24. Loushine BA, Bryan TE, Looney SW, Gillen BM, Loushine RJ, Weller RN, et al. Setting properties and cytotoxicity evaluation of a premixed bioceramic root canal sealer. J Endod. 2011;37:673–7.

25. Xuereb M, Vella P, Damidot D, Sammut CV, Camilleri J. In situ assessment of the setting of tricalcium silicate-based sealers using a dentin pressure model. J Endod. 2015;41:111–24.

26. Ghoneim AG, Lutfy RA, Sabet NE, Fayyad DM. Resistance to fracture of roots obturated with novel canal-filling systems. J Endod. 2011;37:1590–2.

27. Donnermeyer D, Bürklein S, Dammaschke T, Schäfer E. Endodontic sealers based on calcium silicates: a systematic review. Odontology. 2019;107:421–36.

28. Lee JK, Kim S, Lee S, Kim H-C, Kim E. In vitro comparison of biocompatibility of calcium silicate-based root canal sealers. Materials (Basel). 2019;12:2411. https://doi.org/10.3390/ma12152411.

29. Chen B, Haapasalo M, Mobuchon C, Li X, Ma J, Shen Y. Cytotoxicity and the effect of temperature on physical properties and chemical composition of a new calcium silicate–based root canal sealer. J Endod. 2020;46:531–8.

30. Oltra E, Cox TC, LaCourse MR, Johnson JD, Paranjpe A. Retreatability of two endodontic sealers, EndoSequence BC Sealer and AH Plus: a micro-computed tomographic comparison. Restor Dent Endod. 2017;42:19.

31. Heran J, Khalid S, Albaaj F, Tomson PL, Camilleri J. The single cone obturation technique with a modified warm filler. J Dent. 2019;89:103181.

32. Camilleri J. Sealers and warm gutta-percha obturation techniques. J Endod. 2015;41:72–8.

33. Duarte MAH, Marciano MA, Vivan RR, Tanomaru Filho M, Tanomaru JMG, Camilleri J. Tricalcium silicate-based cements: properties and modifications. Braz Oral Res. 2018;32:111–8.

34. http://media.brasselerusa.com/userfiles/IFU%2CManuals%2CBrochures/B_5019_ENG_HiFlow%20NPR.pdf.

35. Dammaschke T. Sealer auf Kalzium-silikatbasis. Der Freie Zahnarzt. 2020;64:64–71.

36. http://www.angelusdental.com/img/arquivos/3823_10503823_0321052018_bio_c_sealer_bula_fechado.pdf.

37. López-García S, Lozano A, García-Bernal D, Forner L, Llena C, Guerrero-Gironés J, et al. Biological effects of new hydraulic materials on human periodontal ligament stem cells. J Clin Med. 2019;8:1216. https://doi.org/10.3390/jcm8081216.

38. Reszka P, Nowicka A, Lipski M, Dura W, Droździk A, Woźniak K. A comparative chemical study of calcium

silicate-containing and epoxy resin-based root canal sealers. Biomed Res Int. 2016;2016:9808432. https://doi.org/10.1155/2016/9808432.

39. Olcay K, Taşli PN, Güven EP, Ülker GMY, Öğüt EE, Çiftçioğlu E, et al. Effect of a novel bioceramic root canal sealer on the angiogenesis-enhancing potential of assorted human odontogenic stem cells compared with principal tricalcium silicate-based cements. J Appl Oral Sci. 2020;28:e20190215. https://doi.org/10.1590/1678-7757-2019-0215.

40. https://www.meta-europe.com/en/produkt/ceraseal/.

41. Komabayashi T, Colmenar D, Cvach N, Bhat A, Primus C, Imai Y. Comprehensive review of current endodontic sealers. Dent Mater J. 2020; https://doi.org/10.4012/dmj.2019-288.

42. López-García S, Myong-Hyun B, Lozano A, García-Bernal D, Forner L, Llena C, et al. Cytocompatibility, bioactivity potential, and ion release of three pre-mixed calcium silicate-based sealers. Clin Oral Investig. 2020;24:1749. https://doi.org/10.1007/s00784-019-03036-2.

43. Colombo M, Poggio C, Dagna A, Meravini M-V, Riva P, Trovati F, et al. Biological and physico-chemical properties of new root canal sealers. J Clin Exp Dent. 2018;10:120–6.

44. Camps J, Jeanneau C, El Ayachi I, Laurent P, About I. Bioactivity of a calcium silicate-based endodontic cement (BioRoot RCS): interactions with human periodontal ligament cells in vitro. J Endod. 2015;41:1469–73.

45. Dimitrova-Nakov S, Uzunoglu E, Ardila-Osorio H, Baudry A, Richard G, Kellermann O, et al. In vitro bioactivity of Bioroot™ RCS, via A4 mouse pulpal stem cells. Dent Mater. 2015;31:1290–7.

46. Prüllage RK, Urban K, Schäfer E, Dammaschke T. Material properties of a tricalcium silicate–containing, a mineral trioxide aggregate–containing, and an epoxy resin–based root canal sealer. J Endod. 2016;42:1784–8.

47. Arias-Moliz MT, Camilleri J. The effect of the final irrigant on the antimicrobial activity of root canal sealers. J Dent. 2016;52:30–6.

48. https://www.septodont.ie/sites/ie/files/2016-11/BioRoot-brochure-UK_0.pdf.

49. Prati C, Gandolfi MG. Calcium silicate bioactive cements: biological perspectives and clinical applications. Dent Mater. 2015;31:351–70.

50. Tomson RME, Polycarpou N, Tomson PL. Contemporary obturation of the root canal system. Br Dent J. 2014;216:315–22.

51. Cailleteau JG. Prevalence of teaching apical patency and various instrumentation and obturation techniques in United States dental schools. J Endod. 1997;23:394–6.

52. Siboni F, Taddei P, Zamparini F, Prati C, Gandolfi MG. Properties of BioRoot RCS, a tricalcium silicate endodontic sealer modified with povidone and polycarboxylate. Int Endod J. 2017;50(Suppl 2):120–36.

53. Dawood AE, Parashos P, Wong RHK, Reynolds EC, Manton DJ. Calcium silicate-based cements:

composition, properties, and clinical applications. J Investig Clin Dent. 2017;8(2) https://doi.org/10.1111/jicd.12195.

54. Gordon MPJ, Love RM, Chandler NP. An evaluation of .06 tapered gutta-percha cones for filling of .06 taper prepared curved root canals. Int Endod J. 2005;38:87–96.

55. Romania C, Beltes P, Boutsioukis C, Dandakis C. Ex-vivo area-metric analysis of root canal obturation using gutta-percha cones of different taper. Int Endod J. 2009;42:491–8.

56. Shahi S, Zand V, Oskoee SS, Abdolrahimi M, Rahnema AH. An in vitro study of the effect of spreader penetration depth on apical microleakage. J Oral Sci. 2007;49:283–6.

57. Allison DA, Michelich RJ, Walton RE. The influence of master cone adaptation on the quality of the apical seal. J Endod. 1981;7:61–5.

58. Schmidt KJ, Walker TL, Johnson JD, Nicoll BK. Comparison of nickel-titanium and stainless-steel spreader penetration and accessory cone fit in curved canals. J Endod. 2000;26:42–4.

59. Berry KA, Loushine RJ, Primack PD, Runyan DA. Nickel-titanium versus stainless-steel finger spreaders in curved canals. J Endod. 1998;24:752–4.

60. Tanomaru-Filho M, Trindade DVB, De Almeida LT, Espir CG, Bonetti-Filho I, Guerreiro-Tanomaru JM. Effect of ProTaper and Reciproc preparation and gutta-percha cone on cold lateral compaction. J Conserv Dent. 2016;19:410–3.

61. Mazotti D, Sivieri-Araújo G, Berbert FLCV, Bonetti-Filho I. In vitro evaluation of the obturation ability, adaptation and compaction of gutta-percha in the root canal system employing different filling techniques. Acta Odontol Latinoam. 2008;21:3–9.

62. Viapiana R, Guerreiro-Tanomaru JM, Tanomaru-Filho M, Camilleri J. Investigation of the effect of sealer use on the heat generated at the external root surface during root canal obturation using warm vertical compaction technique with system b heat source. J Endod. 2014;40:555–61.

63. Viapiana R, Moinzadeh AT, Camilleri L, Wesselink PR, Tanomaru Filho M, Camilleri J. Porosity and sealing ability of root fillings with gutta-percha and BioRoot RCS or AH Plus sealers. Evaluation by three ex vivo methods. Int Endod J. 2016;49:774–82.

64. Nasseh AA, Brave D. Using a bioceramic sealer in conjunction with vertical condensation. Endod Prac. 2015;8:16–20.

65. Buchanan S. Warm gutta-percha obturation with BC HiFlow™ Sealer. Endod Prac. 2018;11:32–5.

66. Koch K, Brave D, Nasseh AA. A review of bioceramic technology in endodontics. Roots. 2013;1:6–13.

67. Germain S, Meetu K, Issam K, Alfred N, Carla Z. Impact of the root canal taper on the apical adaptability of sealers used in a single-cone technique: a micro-computed tomography study. J Contemp Dent Pract. 2018;19:808–15.

68. Celikten B, Uzuntas CF, Orhan AI, Orhan K, Tufenkci P, Kursun S, et al. Evaluation of root canal sealer fill-

ing quality using a single-cone technique in oval shaped canals: an in vitro Micro-CT study. Scanning. 2016;38:133–40.

69. Drukteinis S, Peciuliene V, Shemesh H, Tusas P, Bendinskaite R. Porosity distribution in apically perforated curved root canals filled with two different calcium silicate based materials and techniques: a micro-computed tomography study. Materials (Basel). 2019;12:1729. https://doi.org/10.3390/ma12111729.

70. Moinzadeh AT, Zerbst W, Boutsioukis C, Shemesh H, Zaslansky P. Porosity distribution in root canals filled with gutta percha and calcium silicate cement. Dent Mater. 2015;31:1100–8.

71. Pérez Heredia M, Clavero González J, Ferrer Luque CM, González Rodríguez MP. Apical seal comparison of low-temperature thermoplasticized gutta-percha technique and lateral condensation with two different master cones. Med Oral Patol Oral Cir Bucal. 2007;12:175–9.

72. de Figueiredo FED, Lima LF, Oliveira LS, Ribeiro MA, Correa MB, Brito-Junior M, et al. Effectiveness of a reciprocating single file, single cone endodontic treatment approach: a randomized controlled pragmatic clinical trial. Clin Oral Investig. 2019; https://doi.org/10.1007/s00784-019-03077-7.

73. Kakoura F, Pantelidou O. Retreatability of root canals filled with Gutta percha and a novel bioceramic sealer: a scanning electron microscopy study. J Conserv Dent. 2018;21:632–6.

74. Ersev H, Yilmaz B, Dinçol ME, Dağlaroğlu R. The efficacy of ProTaper Universal rotary retreatment instrumentation to remove single gutta-percha cones cemented with several endodontic sealers. Int Endod J. 2012;45:756–62.

Bioceramic Materials for Management of Endodontic Complications

Saulius Drukteinis

1 Introduction

Prior to the introduction of mineral trioxide aggregate (MTA), the success rates of perforation repair were relatively low due to poor biocompatibility, sealing ability, high cytotoxicity, and hydrophobic properties of the used materials [1]. MTA has changed existing standards in the management of endodontic complications, vital pulp therapy, and regenerative endodontic procedures. However, MTA has a number of limitations, such as problems with mixing, long setting time, difficult handling characteristics and complicated delivery of the material, discoloration of the tooth structure, and the presence of the toxic elements, making the use of this material challenging for many clinicians [2, 3].

During the last decade, the modified hydraulic calcium silicate–based materials for use as root canal sealers, fillers, or root repair materials were introduced to the market [4, 5]. Modifications of the original MTA improved physicochemical, biological properties, and facilitated clinical applicability [6, 7]. The currently available materials are launched as flowable pastes or solid-putty consistency materials. The main biological properties of these materials are quite similar, while the main differences are related to the handling characteristics and application indications [8].

2 Materials Used for Management of Endodontic Complications

There is a wide range of materials available for management of endodontic complications including flowable materials that are launched as premixed and ready-to-use pastes or powder/liquid formulations. Some materials are only suggested to be used as root repair materials in conjunction with different application techniques, while other materials are proposed as sealers or biological fillers and can be used for root canal obturation as well as management of endodontic complications and root repair. The main advantages of flowable hydraulic calcium silicate–based materials are easy manipulation and clinical applicability [8, 9].

2.1 iRoot®BP, EndoSequence® BC RRM™, and TotalFill® BC RRM™ Paste

iRoot®BP, EndoSequence® BC RRM™, and TotalFill® BC RRM™ were the first paste-type and ready-to-use premixed hydraulic calcium silicate–based materials developed for root repair and surgical applications [10, 11] (Fig. 1a). These

S. Drukteinis (✉)
Institute of Dentistry, Vilnius University,
Vilnius, Lithuania

© Springer Nature Switzerland AG 2021
S. Drukteinis, J. Camilleri (eds.), *Bioceramic Materials in Clinical Endodontics*,
https://doi.org/10.1007/978-3-030-58170-1_6

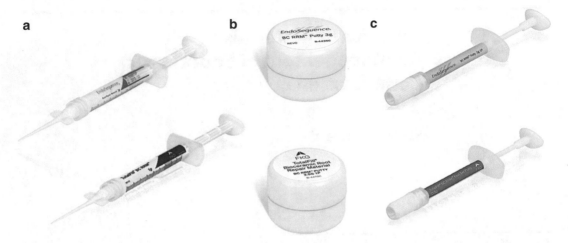

Fig. 1 Different formulations of EndoSequence® BC RRM™ (*upper row*) and TotalFill® BC RRM™ (*lower row*) root repair materials: paste (**a**), putty (**b**), and fast set putty (**c**)

materials are sold under different brand labels; however, they have identical chemical composition, possesses the same physical, biological properties, handling characteristics, and are equally clinically effective [10, 12]. Materials do not shrink in wet environment are radiopaque, aluminum-free and based on a calcium silicate composition, which requires the presence of water to set and harden. The primary difference between RRM paste and BC sealer is that RRM paste contains more filler particles, is more viscous, and has different radiopacifier [9, 11, 13]. These materials are available as root repair pastes in preloaded syringes. The preloaded syringe also has flexible intracanal tips that facilitate its placement in clinical situations. According to the manufacturer's instructions, they have a working time of 30 min and a setting reaction initiated by moisture with a final set achieved approximately within 4 h and is highly dependable on the moisture inside the root canals. The amount of moisture necessary to complete the setting reaction is naturally present in the dentin tubules. Therefore, it is not needed to add moisture in the root canal before placing these materials; however, the root canals should not be excessively desiccated (for example, using alcohol). The indications for use include repair of root perforation, repair of root resorption, root-end (retrograde) filling, apexification, and pulp capping [14, 15].

2.2 iRoot®BP Plus, EndoSequence® BC RRM™, and TotalFill® BC RRM™ Putty

All these materials are convenient ready-to-use white hydraulic premixed putty-type materials developed for permanent repair of large and more easily accessible perforations, resorptions, apexification, and retrofilling [16]. Materials come in the form of premixed condensable putty; their consistency is slightly thicker and more malleable than RRM pastes [17].

As their original formulations, putty materials are radiopaque and aluminum-free materials based on a calcium silicate composition, which requires the presence of water to set and harden [11]. Materials do not shrink during setting and demonstrate excellent physical properties. Their major inorganic components include C_3S, C_2S, and calcium phosphates [18]. Because the materials are premixed with nonaqueous but water-miscible carriers, they do not set during storage and hardens only on exposure to a wet environment [19]. Similar to the paste, the RRM Putty working time is more than 30 min and setting time is 4 h [20]. EndoSequence® BC RRM™ and TotalFill® BC RRM™ Putty are packaged in a preloaded jar [15] (Fig. 1b), while iRoot®BP Plus can be packed in a jar or syringe (Fig. 2a).

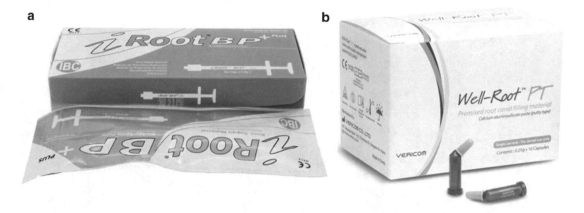

Fig. 2 The iRoot®BP Plus (**a**) and Well-Root™ PT (**b**) putty-type hydraulic calcium silicate–based materials for repair procedures and management of endodontic complications

2.3 iRoot®FS, EndoSequence® BC RRM™, and TotalFill® BC RRM™ Fast Set Putty

iRoot®FS, EndoSequence® BC RRM™, and TotalFill® BC RRM™ Fast Set Putty are modifications of original formulations of the flowable RRM pastes [10, 15]. These materials have the same properties and radiopacity, but their chemical composition differs slightly, which enables materials to harden approximately in 20 min [12, 13]. Due to the accelerated hydration reaction and reduced setting time, materials are extremely resistant to washout, which makes them superior in some specific clinical situations [21].

As their original formulations, these materials are ready to use and EndoSequence® BC RRM™ and TotalFill® BC RRM™ are packed in Sanidose™ syringes (Fig. 1c). The ideal consistency, malleable, and ease of manipulation make these materials usable for various clinical applications [11]. Main clinical advantages are high biocompatibility, bioactivity, and osteogenic potential [22, 23]. Fast set putties possess antibacterial activity, high alkalinity (up to 12 pH) are hydrophilic and do not cause significant discoloration of the hard tissue of the teeth [10, 24].

2.4 Well-Root™ PT

Well-Root™ PT (Vericom, Gangwon-Do, Korea) (Fig. 3b) is a ready to use, premixed, bioceramic paste developed for pulp capping, permanent root canal repair, and surgical applications. It is an insoluble and radiopaque material based on a calcium aluminosilicate composition, which requires the presence of water to set and harden [9]. Well-Root™ PT does not shrink during setting and demonstrates excellent physical and biological properties [25, 26]. It has been shown that material does not create an inflammatory response, promotes mineralization, and demonstrates bioactivity [9]. Some studies using EDS microanalysis, among other elements, detected peaks for sodium, magnesium, aluminum, and titanium in the material [25]. However, the clinical implication of heavy metals contained in Well-Root needs to be investigated [27]. Well-Root™ PT is supplied in packs of 10 × 0.25 g capsules and can be delivered to the application site using a special gun (Fig. 2b).

2.5 Biodentine®

Biodentine® is manufactured by Septodont (Saint-Maur-de-Fosses Cedex, France) and is composed of tricalcium silicate, calcium carbonate, and zirconium oxide as the radiopacifier, while its liquid form contains calcium chloride as the setting accelerator and water-reducing agent. Biodentine® has been launched as a bioactive dentin substitute with the mechanical properties similar to the sound dentin and can replace it both in the crown and in the root [28, 29].

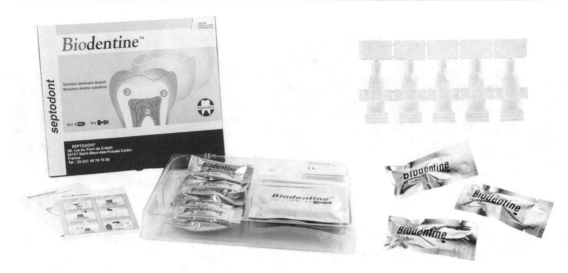

Fig. 3 The package of the Biodentine® contains single-dose powder capsules and vials with a liquid

According to the manufacturer, the "Active Biosilicate Technology®" used to produce Biodentine® ensures the purity of tricalcium silicate, which is what makes this material different from the MTA, which is based on the Portland cement, containing low concentrations of different metal impurities [30, 31]. However, studies have found remains of arsenic, lead and chromium in Biodentine®, but since the release in the physiological solution is minimal, they have been considered safe [32]. Biodentine® comes as a capsule containing powder and a liquid contained in a vial (Fig. 3). According to the mixing instructions, the five drops of the liquid should be squeezed into the capsule and then mixed in an amalgamator for 30 s at a speed of 4000–4200 rotations/min. After mixing, the capsule should be opened and the material's consistency checked. If a thicker consistency is preferred, it is recommended to wait for 30 s to 1 min before checking again [33].

According to the manufacturer, the initial material's setting time is 12 min and is much shorter compared to MTA [34]. From the clinical point of view, it is very important to isolate the operating field during the placement of Biodentine® properly for these 12 min, as water or fluid contamination slows the setting of the material. It has been claimed that the faster setting of the material is related to the smaller size

of the powder particles and a greater reaction area, subsequently. Meanwhile, the calcium chloride in the liquid is a strong accelerator of the setting reaction in Biodentine®, while the presence of calcium carbonate powder increases the hydration reaction of the material [35, 36]. The water-soluble polymer plays an essential role to increase powder density, as the smaller amount of the water is required to obtain the plasticized consistency of the material [31]. Finally, in Biodentine®, the zirconium oxide is added as a radiopacifier, and this is another important difference with MTA, where radiopacity is given by bismuth oxide [37, 38].

3 Temporary Bioceramic–Based Root Canal Dressing Materials

The temporary antibacterial root canal dressing materials are widely used during the endodontic treatment of the teeth with pulp necrosis and apical periodontitis as well as management of endodontic complications [39]. The calcium hydroxide was the material of choice for the interappointment root canal filling used to maximize the root canal disinfection [40–42]. The BIO-C® TEMP is the first ready-to-use bioceramic-based paste for intracanal dressing (Fig. 4). According to the manufacturer, the

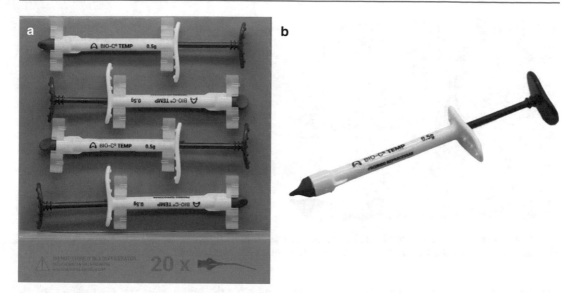

Fig. 4 The package (**a**) and the syringe (**b**) of the first temporary bioceramic-based root canal dressing material BIO-C® TEMP

material is recommended to use as a substitute for conventional calcium hydroxide dressing [43]. The indications for use are intracanal dressing for endodontic treatment in teeth with pulp necrosis and retreatments—intracanal dressing in teeth with perforations, external and internal resorptions, prior to the use of root repair materials—for the apexification procedures.

The composition of the material is calcium silicates, calcium aluminate, calcium oxide, calcium tungstate, and titanium oxide. The material is biocompatible and ready for use, has high alkalinity (pH is 12 ± 1), and radiopacity (9 mm of the aluminum) [43]. The paste is launched in 0.5 g syringes and can be delivered into the root canal via plastic tip cannula, attached to the syringe as the majority of the premixed bioceramic materials.

Before application, the root canal should be irrigated using standard protocols and dried with absorbent paper points. It is recommended to discard the material at the beginning of the syringe, as it may be a little hard. After connection of the applicator tip to the syringe, the tip should be inserted up to 1–2 mm from the established working length. BIO-C® TEMP should be applied through gradual retraction of the syringe to obtain a complete filling of the canals. Any excess of the

paste should be removed from the pulp chamber and temporary filling material placed into endodontic access. The final removal of BIO-C® TEMP before root canal obturation should be performed using sodium hypochlorite and 17% EDTA solution subsequently, which is recommended to activate with an ultrasonic tip in three cycles of 10 s.

It should be mentioned that the product is sensitive to moisture, so the packaging should be properly closed with adequate pressure to prevent dryness. The paste should not be stored in the refrigerator. According to the manufacturer, the paste is easily washable out from the root canals, and the additional irrigation with citric acid is not necessary. It is advantageous in comparison to conventional calcium hydroxide paste, which is difficult to remove from the root canal system.

4 Apexification Procedures

The apexification procedure is performed when the pulp of the tooth with incompletely developed root becomes necrotic, and regenerative treatment procedures are not indicated or possible [44]. The main problems that face clinicians with immature permanent teeth are complicated

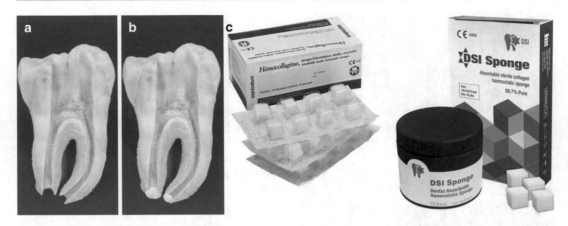

Fig. 5 Immature roots of a mandibular molar with a wide-open apices (**a**). The apical matrix barrier is usually created (**b**) using collagen or hemostatic material (**c**), to prevent extrusion of repair materials

cleaning-shaping and obturation procedures due to the thin root walls and lack of apical barrier [44, 45]. The walls of undeveloped roots are usually thin and very prone to fractures; therefore, mechanical preparation should be performed using minimally invasive techniques [46]. Meanwhile, there is a high risk to extrude the irrigants and obturation materials into periapical tissues because the mineralized apical barrier is absent [47] (Fig. 5a).

Calcium hydroxide has been the material of choice for multiple-visit apexification procedure for a few decades with acceptable success rates [48]. However, the compromised coronal seal between visits and possible recontamination, as well as increased risks of the fracture of the root and crown, were the main clinical concerns, decreasing the success rate of the apexification [48]. For these reasons, the single- or two-appointment apexification using MTA has been introduced and widely used for many years with a very high clinical success rate [49]. However, drawbacks of mixing and hardening, long setting time, difficult handling characteristics and complicated delivery of the material, discoloration of the tooth hard tissues, and the presence of the toxic elements made the use of this material challenging for many clinicians [16].

During the last decade, the hydraulic calcium silicate–based materials were used for apexification procedures with equal success as original MTA [14, 50]. The improved physicochemical

and biological properties, easier clinical applicability, and no effect on the color of the hard tissues of the tooth make these materials superior to the original Portland cement–based MTA [6, 47]. The semi-solid hydraulic calcium silicate–based materials like Biodentine®, iRoot®BP Plus, EndoSequence® BC RRM™, and TotalFill® BC RRM™ Putty were used as apical plugs in the management of the open apices [13, 51]. The clinical procedure is very similar to the technique when the MTA is used as an apical plug. However, before the placement of the material, the obturation technique should be considered by the clinician. These materials can be used just as an apical 4–6 mm plugs [52]; the whole root canal up to the orifice can be filled, or the whole root canal and an endodontic access-tooth crown can be filled and restored [13]. If the endodontic access is filled, the materials are used as a dentine substitute, expecting to reinforce tooth crown and root. It has been shown that complete root canal and endodontic access filling with Biodentine®, as a dentine substitute, increased the tooth resistance to the fractures, longevity, and survival rates [53, 54].

Due to the wide foraminal opening, the apexification procedure often requires placement of the matrix or apical barrier, to prevent or minimize the extrusion of the hydraulic calcium silicate–based materials periapically (Fig. 5b). Despite the excellent biological properties and biocompatibility of these materials, their extrusion is not recommended and should be avoided [47, 50, 55]. A number of the materials have been recommended to be used as a matrix; however, the hemostatic sponges or collagen are the most popular [45, 47, 56] (Fig. 5c). The matrix materials can be delivered to the apical-periapical region via the prepared root canal using pre-fitted gutta-percha plugger using gentle condensation of the barrier material apically. These materials are very well tolerated by periapical tissues and are resorbed within a few days [45, 56]. They perform not only as a mechanical barrier but also as a moisture control, as they protect the hydraulic calcium silicate–based materials from the contamination with tissue fluids or blood and possible washout [51].

After isolation of the tooth with a rubber dam and endo access opening, the root canal is prepared using suitable endodontic instruments and appropriate irrigants (Fig. 6a). After preparation, the root canal should be dried with paper points; however, overdrying should be avoided. The apical matrix-barrier using collagen should be established as described previously (Fig. 6b). If the material used as an apical plug is requiring mixing prior to its application (for example, Biodentine®), it should be done according to the manufacturer's recommendations. No specified preparations are needed for the premixed putty-type hydraulic calcium silicate–based materials [11]. Materials are delivered to the root canal

using a suitable instrument and gently condensed with a pre-fitted plugger (Fig. 6c). The indirect sonic or ultrasonic agitation of the materials has been recommended to decrease the porosity and increase the sealability of the materials [57, 58]. However, there is a lack of solid and sufficient scientific background to support this recommendation. The X-ray should be taken after the procedure to check that the material is homogeneous and correctly positioned. If the voids in the material or inadequate length of the apical plug are detected, additional condensation should be applied, and new X-ray should be taken.

Recently, the Type 5 fast set putty materials such as iRoot®FS, EndoSequence® BC RRM™, and TotalFill® BC RRM™ Fast Set Putty were introduced and successfully used as apical plugs during apexification procedures [13]. The short setting time allows the completion of the treatment procedure in a single visit, which is advantageous in comparison to regular putty materials and is quite similar to the procedure using Biodentine® [13].

If the hydraulic calcium silicate–based materials are used just as apical plugs, the rest of the root canal should be obturated with thermoplastic gutta-percha and sealer. Usually, it is performed during the next visit, as the long setting time of the materials does not allow to finish whole apexification procedure at the single appointment. After initial setting of apical plugs, the

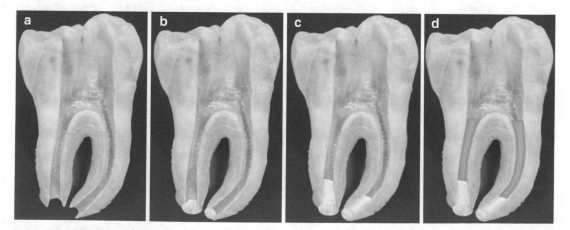

Fig. 6 Two-appointment apexification procedure using Biodentine® or puty-type RRM. At the first visit, open apices (**a**) are isolated with barrier material (**b**), and

4–6 mm of a root repair material as an apical plug is placed (**c**). The remaining root canals are obturated at the second visit with gutta-percha and the sealer (**d**)

empty root canal space can be filled with inject-able calcium hydroxide paste, and the temporary filling material should be placed. During the sec-ond visit, the tooth is reopened under aseptic con-ditions, and the root canal obturated with gutta-percha and sealer (Fig. 6d).

The tooth crown should be restored with a per-manent restoration. If the entire root canal has obturated with the hydraulic calcium silicate–based material, just endodontic access isolation with a temporary filling material is needed at the first appointment, and the final restoration is placed during the second visit.

As it was mentioned before, to maximize the reinforcement capabilities of the condensable hydraulic calcium silicate–based materials and replace radicular, cervical, and coronal dentine, it was suggested to use Biodentine® or putty-type RRM to fill entire canal of the undeveloped root as well as entire endodontic access [53]. The few superficial millimeters of the set hydraulic cal-cium silicate–based material can be replaced with composite after 3–6 months during the fol-low-up appointment [59] (Fig. 7).

Despite the fact that root canals of undevel-oped roots usually are very wide, and the apical part of the canal is easily accessible under or sometimes even without magnification, some clinical situations can still be challenging. Those difficulties usually are related to multirooted teeth with significant root curvatures. In these situations, the paste-type root repair materials like iRoot®BP, EndoSequence® BC RRM™, and TotalFill® BC RRM™ Paste can be successfully used in conjunction with injection technique. These materials can be used during the two-visit apexification procedure as an apical 4–6 mm plugs, a subsequentially obturating root canal with gutta-percha and sealer (Fig. 8).

Also, these RRM pastes can be used for the single-visit apexification procedure, when the entire root canal is filled with the paste at the level of the orifices (Fig. 9).

For both techniques, the clinical steps of isola-tion, cleaning-shaping as well as final crown res-toration are identical to these, when putty-type materials are used and were described before.

5 Perforation Repair

Iatrogenic errors, such as root canal transporta-tions, ledging, zipping, and others, can lead to uncontrolled and accidental root perforations. The risk of perforations significantly increases during endodontic retreatment procedures [60, 61]. Visualization of the perforation area is a very important factor leading to the success of the

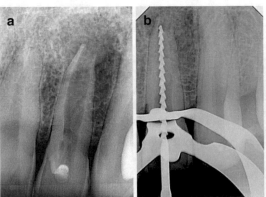
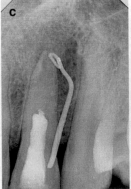
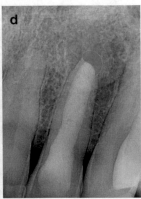

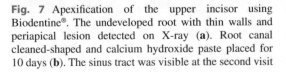

Fig. 7 Apexification of the upper incisor using Biodentine®. The undeveloped root with thin walls and periapical lesion detected on X-ray (**a**). Root canal cleaned-shaped and calcium hydroxide paste placed for 10 days (**b**). The sinus tract was visible at the second visit (**c**); root canal was recleaned and calcium hydroxide paste replaced. No complaints or clinical signs were detected at the third visit; the apical barrier was created using Hemocollagene and root canal, and endo access were filled with Biodentine® (**d**)

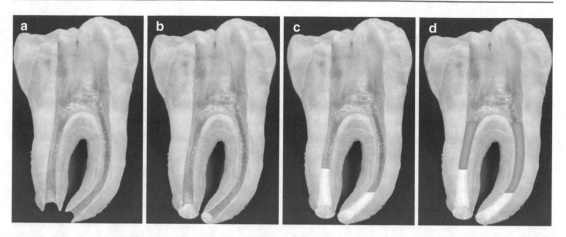

Fig. 8 Two-appointment apexification procedure using injectable RRM paste. At the first visit, open apices (**a**) are isolated with barrier material (**b**), and 4–6 mm of a flow- able root repair material as an apical plug is placed (**c**). The remaining root canals are obturated at the second visit with gutta-percha and the sealer (**d**)

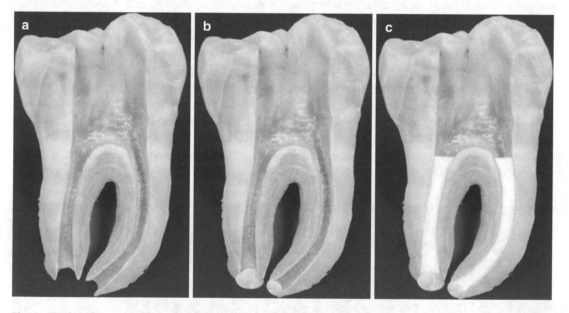

Fig. 9 Single-visit apexification procedure using injectable RRM paste, filling entire canals of undeveloped roots. Open apices (**a**) are isolated with a barrier material (**b**) and entire root canals obturated with a flowable RRM paste (**c**)

treatment; however, direct observation of perfo- rations beyond the curvature of the root canal is limited even if a dental microscope is used [62]. It leads to the complicated delivery of repair material, lack of appropriate control during con- densation, and, as a consequence, poor apical seal [63].

5.1 Definition, Etiology, and Clinical Manifestation

Perforations are defined as communication between the root canal system and the periodon- tal tissues [64]. They can be caused by the patho- logical process, like caries or resorption, or can be created iatrogenically during endodontic treatment or especially retreatment (zip, strip, furcation perforations) as well as during restoration of endodontically treated teeth (for example, post preparation perforation). It has been shown that 53% of all perforations occur during prosthetic and 47% during endodontic treatment procedures [2]. When perforation occurs, the inflammatory reaction in the periodontal tissues starts and progresses if the perforation is not managed using biocompatible materials [65]. The inflammation is caused by both mechanical trauma with endodontic instruments or burs and extrusion of the debris, microorganisms, and their byproducts to the perforation site [64].

It has been concluded that the perforation should be immediately sealed after identification as delayed sealing is directly related to the worse prognosis or even the loss of the tooth [64]. Sometimes, the treatment of the perforations requires a multidisciplinary approach—nonsurgical and surgical procedures are required. From the clinical point of view, the level, position, size–shape, and time of occurring of the perforation are the most critical factors influencing the treatment approach and outcome [1, 61]. Perforations can occur in all thirds of the root,

while the apical and middle-root perforations have a better prognosis in comparison to coronal or furcal perforations [62].

The localization of perforations can be as diverse as possible. They can be located on the buccal or lingual, mesial or distal surfaces of the roots. It has been concluded that the sealing quality mainly depends on the size and shape of the perforation—the bigger size of the perforation, the bigger area of exposed periodontal tissues should be covered and sealed. Usually, the lateral or furcal perforations are oval-shaped or elliptical as they are made with a bur or endodontic instrument crossing the dentin under the angle. However, the cross-sectional configuration and size of apical perforations related to previous transportation, ledging, and over-instrumentation in curved roots are unpredictable [66]. They can vary significantly, depending on the root length, radius, and degree of the curvature (Fig. 10), making the management of these perforations even more complicated.

Apical perforations usually occur as a consequence of inaccurate instrumentation of curved canals, transporting the apical third of the canal and destroying the integrity of the apex. The most crucial aim in this clinical situation is the negoti-

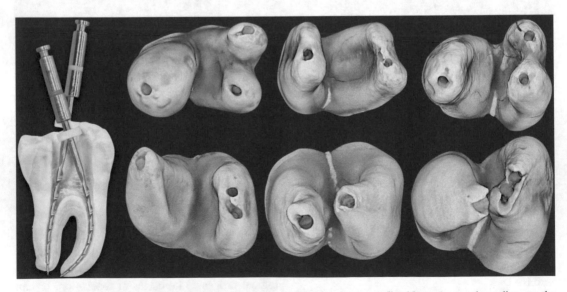

Fig. 10 3D micro-CT reconstructions of the experimentally perforated curved roots of mandibular molars. The cross-sectional diameter and configuration of apical perforations are unpredictable and vary depending on the anatomical features of the roots

ation of the original root canal (using pre-curved hand instruments, copious irrigation, and constant agitation of the irrigants). If the procedure is successful, the original root canal is cleaned, shaped, and obturated, no additional sealing of the perforation is required, especially if it is small, "spot" type perforation. However, this clinical condition is a bit more historical. Nowadays, the majority of the root canals are shaped using engine-driven endodontic instruments. It should be mentioned that if the apex is perforated with a large taper rotary or reciprocating file, the size of the perforation will be much larger than the original size of the instrument. It is related to the significant increase in the diameter of the instrument with every millimeter of its length. If the perforation is made with the same size, but different taper instruments (for example, 0.4, 0.6, 0.7, or 0.8), the perforation diameters will vary significantly. Moreover, the alloy of the instrument is directly related to the perforation size in curved roots, too. All NiTi instruments possess a so-called "shape memory" effect and are trying to straighten in the curved root canals [67]. If perforation occurs and the instrument is rotating beyond the apex, the cross-sectional shape of perforation will become even more oval [68]. Therefore, the CM NiTi instruments do not have any negative straightening effect on the root canals and are less "harmful" if perforations occur [69].

The middle-third perforations usually occur during cleaning and shaping of the canal system or the preparation of a post space using rotary instruments such as Peeso or Largo reamers, Gates Glidden burs, or others [70]. These perforations can occur in all teeth, requiring the metallic or fiber post for crown restoration. To avoid these perforations, the main preoperative factors should be determined before post space preparation: the inclination of the tooth, the individual anatomical features, the curvature and thickness of the root, and the size of the bur [71]. The second type of middle-root perforations is strip perforations, usually occurring on the concave side of the mesial roots of lower or mesiobuccal roots of upper molars [72]. Usually, the excessive amount of the dentin is removed by the operator, due to aggressive instrumentation using rigid stainless steel or big taper endodontic instruments.

Furcal or coronal-third perforations usually occur during endo access preparation in teeth with extensive pulp chamber calcification or different angles of tooth inclination [73]. These perforations can be made by preparing the space for the different types of the post when preoperational risk factors are not considered. The floor of the pulp chamber or coronal-third of the root usually is perforated by the clinician exploring the obliterated orifices of the root canals or losing the anatomical signs. Even the use of the magnification or ultrasonic devices not always guarantee success. If the perforations are not managed immediately, there is an increased risk of the rapid alveolar bone resorption, migration of the epithelium, and periodontal pocket formation [74]. The treatment of these periodontal defects becomes complicated and adversely affects the prognosis and survival of the tooth [75].

The time when perforations occur and when they are sealed is an essential factor for prognostication of the outcome [62]. Perforation causes the inflammatory reaction in the surrounding tissues and prolonged period can cause a substantial breakdown of periodontal tissue, which can complicate the management of old perforations or even cause the tooth loss [74]. It is widely accepted that perforations should be sealed as soon as possible, preferably at the same appointment of their occurrence [64, 75].

5.2 Techniques of the Perforation Repair

The selection of the material to be used for root perforation repair in every clinical situation highly depends on the clinical conditions, such as size and localization of the perforation, the possibility to access the perforation site directly, deliver and manipulate repair material under visual control, and the experience of the operator. If the clinical situation is complicated and not allows the clinician to deliver and condensate cement or putty-type material under appropriate control, it is recommended to use flowable materials. It can be expected that due to the high flowability and penetrability of the hydraulic calcium silicate–based materials, the sealing quality of the difficultly accessible perforation site will be better.

5.2.1 Perforation Repair Using Putty-Type Materials

The Type 5 hydraulic calcium silicate–based root repair materials that are launched as a semi-solid plasticized or putty-type materials are different in their applicability in comparison to MTA cement. These materials are not hard or brittle but rather more plastic [16]. The hydraulic calcium silicate–based root repair materials like a Biodentine® should be mixed before use, while the iRoot®BP Plus, EndoSequence® BC RRM™/TotalFill® BC RRM™ Putty as well as their fast setting formulations iRoot®FS, EndoSequence® BC RRM™/ TotalFill® BC RRM™ Fast Set Putty are pre-mixed and can be used without any additional preparation. It has been shown that some condensation of these materials is needed to achieve homogeneous and voids-free fillings [15, 76]. Thus, preferably the clinicians using these materials for the management of perforations should have appropriate direct visual control to deliver and condensate materials at the perforation site. Clinically, these putty-type condensable materials are recommended to be used for management of all perforations: furcation, coronal, middle or apical, and repair procedure by itself is not very different as it is using MTA cement.

For the repair of furcation perforation, the tooth should be isolated with a rubber dam, endo access opened and disinfected with a sodium hypochlorite, perforation sites visualized, and the size identified [17, 72]. It is recommended to use a collagen or hemostatic material barrier matrix to control bleeding and exudation and prevent the extrusion of repair material into periodontal tissues [75]. The additional attention should be paid to the old perforations, as these are often associated with the bone resorption in the furcation area [74]. Subsequentially, more barrier material can be required to create an adequate matrix in the resorbed bone. Finally, the pulp chamber is gently dried with a dry cotton pellet, and preferable hydraulic calcium silicate–based material is dispensed and condensed in small increments until the perforation is repaired (Fig. 11). Perforation repair and crown restoration can be performed in a single step if fast setting materials are used.

If the root perforation, which can be visualized and well accessed using magnification, repair using putty-type materials is performed, the tooth is isolated with a rubber dam, endo access opened and disinfected, the perforation site is accessed, and size of perforation is identified. Thereafter, the root canal cleaning-shaping procedures should be done in a conventional manner avoiding over-instrumentation or extrusion of irrigants beyond perforation [77]. A root canal should be dried and can be filled with antibacterial dressing material (for example, calcium hydroxide or bioceramic-based paste) for disinfection between visits. If temporary dressing is used, the endo access should be isolated with an intermediate restorative material. At the next visit, the tooth is isolated, endo access reopened, root canal recleaned, dried, and preferable putty-type hydraulic calcium silicate–based material is dispensed over the perforation site using a suitable instrument and condensed with a plugger. The excess material should be removed, root canal filled with calcium hydroxide/bioceramic-based paste and a temporary filling placed. The root canal treatment should be completed at the next visit according to the current recommendations [17].

5.2.2 Perforation Repair Using Flowable Materials and Injection Technique

The direct visualization of the perforation site and control of repair procedures have an important impact on the outcome of the perforation repair [62]. Even if the handling characteristics and clinical applicability of the new fourth and fifth type hydraulic calcium silicate–based putty-type materials are superior to MTA, some clinical challenges still exist. It should be mentioned that even under magnification, the repair

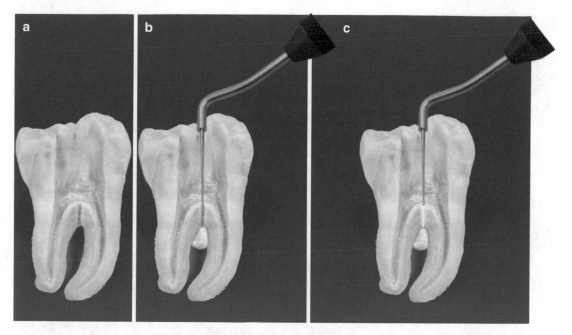

Fig. 11 Furcation perforation of mandibular molar (**a**). The matrix-barrier is created using collagen-based material delivered into the furcation area using pre-fitted plugger, smaller than perforation diameter (**b**). The putty-type hydraulic calcium silicate–based material is delivering to the perforation in small increments and condensed against matrix (**c**)

of the root perforations that are localized in a difficultly accessible sites (for example, apical perforation in curved roots) with a limited direct visibility, the flowable paste-type root repair materials can be superior in comparison to condensable putty-type materials. Another clinical situation, when these paste-type materials can be superior over the condensable hydraulic calcium silicate—based materials are small furcation perforations or perforations in narrow root canals when material delivery even using smallest plugger is not convenient or possible. Moreover, it has been shown that the smaller perforation, the fewer chances that significant bone resorption, and periodontal tissue breakdown will occur [61, 62]. Therefore, the matrix or barrier in case of the small perforation is usually not needed, as the periapical tissue pressure is sufficient to protect from the extrusion of the repair material, especially non-condensable [70, 78] (Fig. 12). If injectable root perforation repair is selected, all clinical steps and procedures before delivering the materials are the same, as described previously.

5.2.3 Perforation Repair Using Single-Cone or Modified Single-Cone Obturation Techniques

The performance of flowable hydraulic calcium silicate—based root repair pastes, as perforation repair materials, is well investigated [11, 15]. However, these materials are quite expensive and often not available in the daily general dental practice. It has been shown that majority of endodontic complications are treated by endodontists instead of general practitioners [79, 80]. However, the root canal obturation using hydraulic calcium silicate–based sealers and single-cone obturation technique is gaining popularity among general dentists [81]. It can be expected that they are familiar with the properties of these sealers and clinical applicability.

Recently. it has been claimed that hydraulic calcium silicate–based sealers such as BioRoot™ RCS, EndoSequence® BC Sealer™, and TotalFill® BC Sealer™ can be used not only as sealers but also as injectable biological fillers, too [82, 83]. Main properties of these materials such

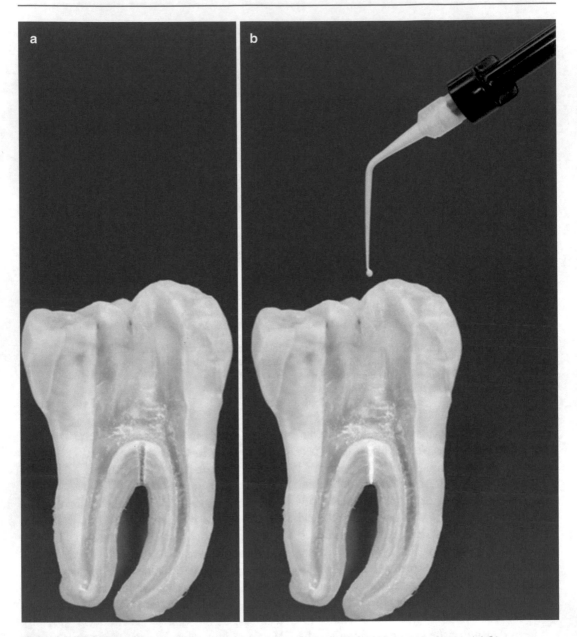

Fig. 12 Small diameter furcation perforation (**a**) can be repaired using injectable root repair material (**b**)

as antimicrobial activity, biocompatibility, and bioactivity are identical to root repair formulations [84]. Thus, these materials can be used as biological fillers in clinical situations, when significant root repair–dentine replacement or root reinforcement is not needed, and when the perforation and communication of the root canal space and periodontal tissues is not extensive [33]. These clinical situations can be an accidental api-

cal root canal transportations and perforations, lateral or strip root perforations, with a limited or difficult accessibility and lack of direct visual control [78].

When the strip or lateral perforation is localized in the middle-apical thirds at the level of the root curve or beyond, but the integrity of the apical constriction is not damaged, there is a possibility to repair existing perforations without any specific repair manipulations or proce- dures. After root canal debridement using copious irrigation with appropriate irrigants and irrigation techniques, canals of perforated roots should be dried and master gutta-percha point pre-fitted. Afterwards, the root canal is filled with flowable hydraulic calcium silicate– based sealer, which in these clinical situations are used as a biological filler, and gutta-percha point is reinserted to the full working length. The superior flowability of the materials and additional hydraulic pressure inside root canal can ensure distribution and penetration of the sealer-filler into the "false canal" and seal the perforation without any additional manipula- tions (Fig. 13).

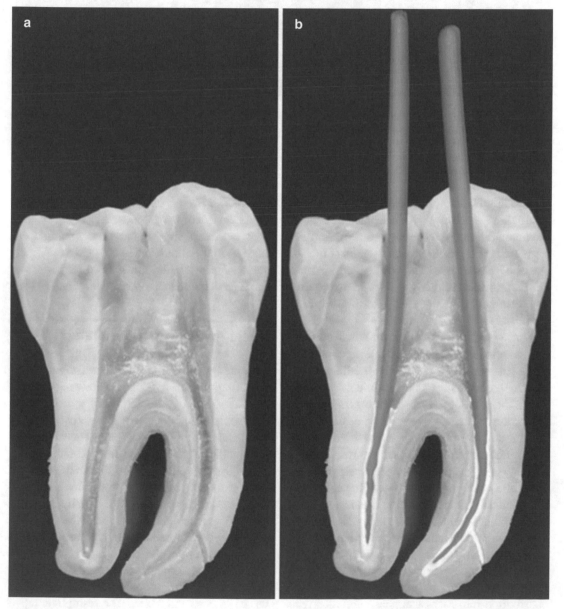

Fig. 13 Small lateral root perforations (**a**) can be man- aged without any specific treatment procedures, if flow- able hydraulic calcium silicate--based material and single-cone technique are used for obturation; high flow- ability and penetrability of the material can ensure accept- able results (**b**)

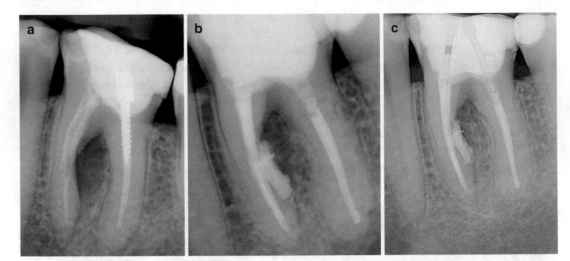

Fig. 14 Management of the strip perforation of the tooth 36, using a modified single-cone obturation technique. Preoperative radiograph shows strip perforation of the mesial root and extensive lesion in the furcation area (**a**). Endodontic retreatment performed using conventional cleaning and shaping protocol and 1-week calcium hydroxide therapy; root canals were obturated with BioRoot™ RCS sealer and single gutta-percha cone (**b**). No clinical symptoms and noticeable healing of the lesion 12 months after endodontic retreatment (**c**)

The single-cone root canal obturation technique can be used by general practitioners for the management of some endodontic complications with acceptable clinical results (Fig. 14). Despite some evidence of success, more clinical investigations are needed to confirm the clinical efficiency of these simplified techniques.

However, if the integrity of the apical constriction is affected, the standard single-cone technique in conjunction with hydraulic calcium silicate–based sealers–fillers should be modified. Using the modified single-cone obturation technique, the master gutta-percha point is selected, pre-fitted at the full working length with a tug-back effect, and cut 2–3 mm shorter than the working length with a sterile scalpel. When hydraulic calcium silicate–based flowable material is delivered into the root canal, and gutta-percha point is reinserted, the apical 2–3 mm are filled with antibacterial, biocompatible, and bioactive material, which comes into direct contact with periodontal tissues (Fig. 15). The gutta-percha point helps to improve the sealer–filler distribution into root canal space and all irregularities. This modified technique can be clinically appealing because it does not require superior handling skills of the clinician nor the direct visual control of the procedure.

It has been shown that this technique can ensure tight, homogeneous, and minimally porous filling of the apical third of perforated curved roots of mandibular molars (Fig. 16) [58].

6 Repair of Resorptive Defects

The etiology of external and internal tooth resorption is multifactorial [85, 86]. They can be caused by pulp necrosis, dental trauma, orthodontic treatment, professional hygiene procedures, or tooth whitening [87, 88]. The treatment modalities significantly depend on the type and localization of the resorption [89]. While small defects of the apical external resorption can be just monitored or internal root resorption usually is not difficult to manage and repair, and the extensive external cervical resorption can be extremely challenging for the clinicians.

Calcium hydroxide as a material of choice for treatment of different resorptions was used until the MTA was introduced for resorption repair [90, 91]. However, previously mentioned drawbacks of these materials, made the hydraulic

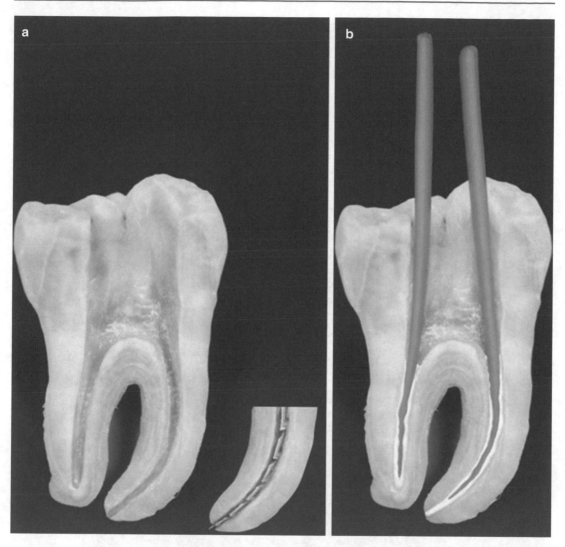

Fig. 15 If accidental apical root perforation is made with a smaller endodontic instrument (**a**), the modified single-cone obturation technique with hydraulic calcium silicate–based sealer-filler can be used for repair (**b**)

calcium silicates very popular for the management of external and internal resorption [15, 92]. Depending on the type of resorptions, they can be repaired using flowable and solid hydraulic calcium silicate–based materials. External apical inflammatory, internal or internal-perforating resorptions can be repaired using all available materials (Fig. 17). While external cervical resorptions preferably should be repaired using fast set type materials, to avoid possible wash out of the material [15, 93, 94].

It has been shown that apical periodontitis with a periapical lesion is very often associated with an extensive external apical inflammatory root resorption, which usually is not visible on conventional radiographs [95, 96]. The resorption usually progresses from the tip of the root towards apical constriction, and after some time crater-type defect on the tip of the root is established, and natural apical stop is disrupted. These resorbed root tips look like undeveloped roots or roots with extensive apical root perforation. If conventional root canal obturation technique with pre-fitted master gutta-percha point is selected, despite the tug-back effect was achieved, there is a risk that some resorbed areas will not be

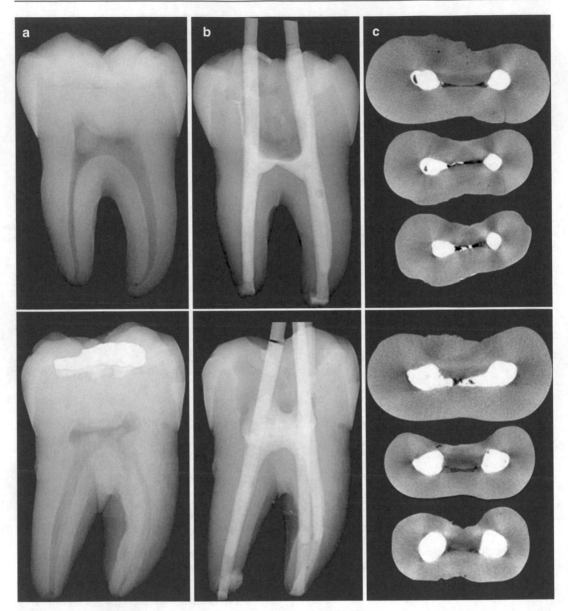

Fig. 16 Mandibular molars before experimental apical perforation of the curved roots (**a**). X-rays of the teeth, after filling of apical perforations root canals with BioRoot™ RCS as a filler and in conjunction with single gutta-percha point, using modified obturation technique (**b**). The cross-sectional images of micro-CT scan at coronal, middle, and apical thirds of the roots (*top to bottom*), demonstrating the homogeneity of the fillings (**c**)

hermetically sealed (Fig. 18). Thus, the clinicians can face a serious problem, which is not detectable neither clinically nor radiographically.

In this case, the injectable hydraulic calcium silicate–based root repair material or previously described modified single-cone obturation technique with a sealer-filler can be used, to fill

1–2 mm of the apical root canal with a hydraulic calcium silicate–based material.

Non-perforating or perforating internal root resorptions can be repaired using a wide range of Type 4 or Type 5 hydraulic calcium silicate–based materials [15]. The treatment preferably should be performed under profound anesthesia and a rubber dam isolation. The root canal should be accessed in a conventional way, while a cleaning and shaping procedures should be accompanied with a copious root canal irrigation with a solution of sodium hypochlorite agitated using sonic or ultrasonic agitation techniques [97]. The root canal and resorption defect should be dried with paper points and filled with calcium hydroxide or temporary bioceramic paste for disinfection between visits. It is recommended to use premixed pastes as these materials are easier to inject into the root canal and fill resorption defect due to the increased flowability of these materials [98]. Meanwhile, the removal of these premixed pastes is easier in comparison to *ex tempore* mixed paste, due to the additives decreasing the adhesion of the materials to the dentin [99]. Afterwards, the access cavity should be filled with temporary cement to protect the temporary root canal filling. At the next visit (usually after

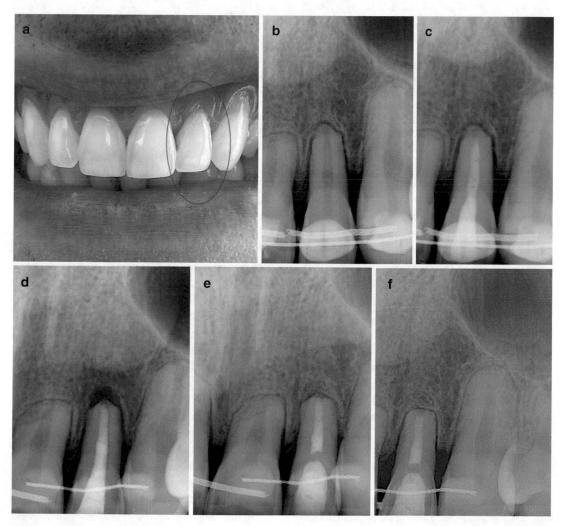

Fig. 17 Clinical (**a**) and radiographic (**b**) view of the tooth 22 2 weeks after trauma. Mild sensitivity on the bitewing and percussion, no reaction to thermal tests were detected. Extensive generalized root resorption after orthodontic treatment was visible. Conventional cleaning and shaping were performed, and premixed calcium hydroxide paste was placed for 1-week (**c**), and replaced for additional 2 weeks, due to some mild discomfort on bitewing and increased periapical radiolucency on the follow-up X-ray (**d**). The tooth was asymptomatic after 2 weeks; the entire root canal was filled with Biodentine®, using Hemocollagene as an apical matrix (**e**). No clinical symptoms or visible changes on X-ray were detected after 6 months follow-up (**f**)

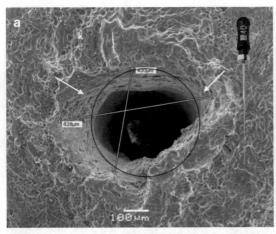 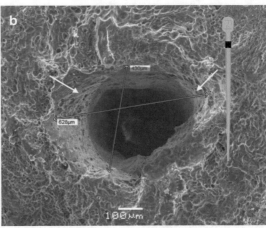

Fig. 18 SEM images of the surface of the tip of the medial root of the mandibular molar, affected by chronic apical periodontitis associated with the periapical lesion. Crater-type external resorption disrupted the integrity of apical constriction, while the root canal cross-sectional configuration is not uniform. If root canal will be enlarged up to file #40 (**a**) and the same size master gutta-percha point will be pre-fitted with a tug-back effect at the full WL (**b**), some resorbed areas—irregularities—(*white rows*) will be filled just with sealer, which potentially can be resorbed, compromising the tight apical seal over the time

1 week), a rubber dam should be placed, the temporary restoration removed, calcium hydroxide or bioceramic paste flushed out using citric acid [100], and root canal recleaned in the same manner as the first visit. Subsequentially, root canal/resorption defect is dried with paper points and filled with the preferable material. If plasticized materials like a Biodentine®, iRoot®BP Plus, EndoSequence® BC RRM™, and TotalFill® BC RRM™ Putty are used, the root canal below the resorption defect is obturated using gutta-percha and sealer. Subsequently, repair materials are delivered over the resorptive defect using a suitable instrument and gently condensed with a plugger. Meanwhile, if the paste-type materials are used, the entire root canal and resorption defect can be filled by injecting these materials. After the filling of the root canal and resorption defect, the X-ray to check that the material is correctly positioned should be taken (Fig. 19). Finally, the temporary filling or permanent restoration should be placed, depending on the clinical situation.

Aggressive and extensive external cervical root resorptions are challenging when they cause significant root damage [85]. However, when extensive resorption defect results in pulpits and subsequently infection of the resorption defect, the endodontic treatment of the tooth in conjunction with surgical repair of the root is the only viable option to save a tooth [101]. However, if external cervical resorption is extensive, the extraction of the tooth can be the only treatment of choice [86]. In cases when direct surgical access with good visualization of the resorption defect can be achieved, the use of fourth or fifth type of hydraulic calcium silicate–based repair materials, which are easy to apply to the site and have demonstrated excellent biocompatibility, bonding, and hydrophilic qualities, nowadays should be the first clinical choice. It has been shown that the use of nanoparticulate premixed fast setting putty formulations can be superior due to decreased risks to be washed out [94]. Long-term follow-up of the healing of the compromised clinical cases of external cervical resorption repair revealed good periodontal tissues healing, acceptable esthetics, and a lack of dentin staining [101, 102].

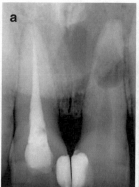
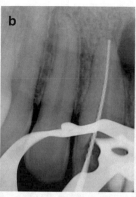
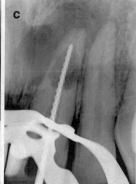
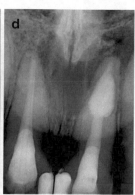

Fig. 19 The perforating internal resorption and lesion of the surrounding tissues of the tooth 21 and apical periodontitis of the tooth 11 (**a**). Endodontic retreatment for tooth 11 and treatment for tooth 21 performed using conventional cleaning and shaping protocol and 1-week calcium hydroxide therapy (**b, c**). The root canal of the tooth 11 was obturated with BioRoot™ RCS sealer in conjunction with a big taper single gutta-percha point; the root canal and resorption defect of the tooth 21 were filled with a TotalFill® BC RRM™ Paste (**d**)

7 Endodontic Surgery Procedures

When endodontic treatment is not successful, and nonsurgical endodontic retreatment fails or is not possible, the endodontic surgery is indicated [103]. However, due to the rapid developments in implant dentistry, the endodontic surgery is becoming less popular in comparison to the tooth replacement with an implant. It should be mentioned that some clinical investigations detected better prognosis of the dental implant in comparison to retreatment procedure; however, well-designed clinical trials demonstrated the opposite—the endodontic retreatment is equally effective treatment option, if not superior [104].

The MTA was a material of choice as a retrograde filling with high clinical success rates [105]. However, due to the drawbacks of MTA, mentioned before, the Type 4 and 5 hydraulic calcium silicate–based root repair materials have become more and more popular and widespread use in endodontic surgery [13, 106]. The current scientific findings indicate that these materials possess superior properties and handling characteristic and provide similar healing rates after endodontic surgery as MTA cement [107, 108] (Fig. 20).

After the exposure and apicoectomy, the 3–5 mm-depth retrograde cavity should be prepared with appropriate ultrasonic tip, keeping the alignment with the long axis of the root, following the direction and the outline contour of the root canal [109, 110]. The retrograde filling material should be prepared and delivered to the cavity using appropriate instruments, such as Lucas curette (Hu-Friedy Mfg. Co., Chicago, IL, USA), MAP System (Produits Dentaires SA, Vevey, Switzerland), or Dovgan applicator (Vista Dental Products, Racine, WI, USA). A biocompatible and bioactive hydraulic calcium silicate–based material is used to create a stable hermetic seal that can prevent the percolation of bacteria or their products between root canal system and periradicular tissues and promote the healing of these tissues. To prevent the washout of the hydraulic calcium silicate–based retrograde materials, the fast setting formulations such as Biodentine®, iRoot®FS, EndoSequence® BC RRM™, and TotalFill® BC RRM™ Fast Set Putty can be superior to the slow setting putty-type materials [111] (Fig. 21). However, if original formulations are used, the surgical wound should not be irrigated, since this can result in dislodgement of the material. The excess of retro filler should be gently removed with a wet sterile cotton gauze before flap reposition and placement of the sutures.

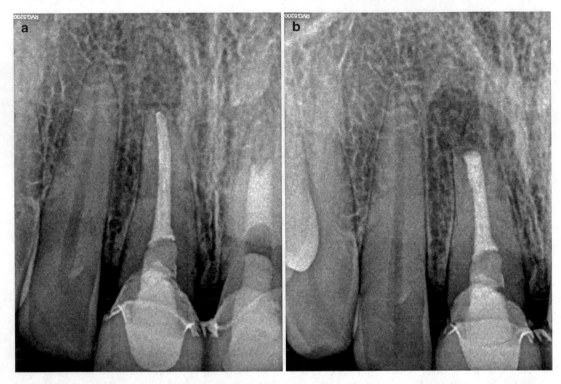

Fig. 20 The successful surgical management of non-healing apical periodontitis. After retreatment and placement of the crown, the clinical and radiographic signs of symptomatic apical periodontitis recovered (**a**). After api-coectomy, root-end preparation was performed using ultrasonic tips, and the retrograde cavity was filled with a TotalFill® BC RRM™ Fast Set Putty (**b**). (*Courtesy Antanas Blazys, DDS*)

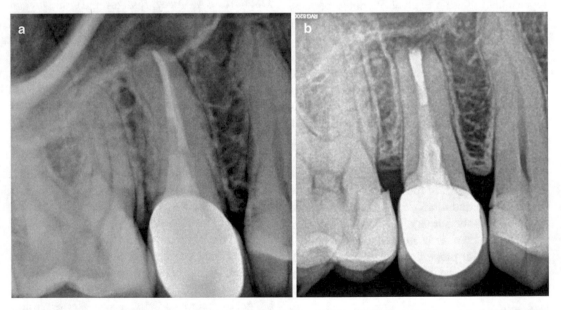

Fig. 21 The clinical symptoms and radiographic signs of apical periodontitis 3 years after endodontic-prosthetic treatment were detected at the day of the patient's visit (**a**). Endodontic surgery was performed, filling the retrograde cavity with a TotalFill® BC RRM™ Fast Set Putty (**b**). CBCT evaluation before surgical intervention revealed the poor quality of primary endodontic treatment and large periapical lesion (**c–f**). (*Courtesy Antanas Blazys, DDS*)

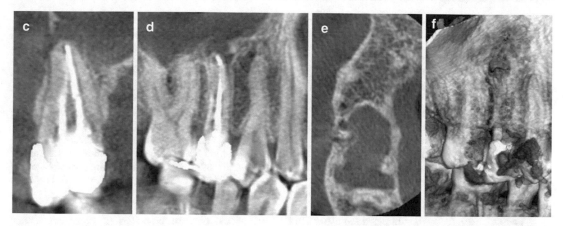

Fig. 21 (continued)

8 Conclusions

Many years ago, MTA has changed existing standards in the management of endodontic complications, vital pulp therapy, or regenerative endodontic procedures. However, the drawbacks of the MTA discussed in this chapter made the use of this material challenging for many clinicians. Recently, the Types 4 and 5 of commercially available hydraulic calcium silicate–based materials have superceded the original MTA and similar formulations as materials of choice for the management of endodontic complications. Nowadays, plasticized, putty-type or paste-type repair hydraulic calcium silicate–based materials are widely researched, and the clinical effectiveness, as well as advantages over Portland cement formulations, are confirmed. The solid scientific background indicates that the newer types of hydraulic calcium silicate–based materials can replace MTA and are the future materials for the management of endodontic complications.

References

1. Siew K, Lee AHC, Cheung GSP. Treatment outcome of repaired root perforation: a systematic review and meta-analysis. J Endod. 2015;41:1795. https://doi.org/10.1016/j.joen.2015.07.007.
2. Clauder T, Shin S-J. Repair of perforations with MTA: clinical applications and mechanisms of action. Endod Top. 2006;15:32. https://doi.org/10.1111/j.1601-1546.2009.00242.x.
3. Parirokh M, Torabinejad M, Dummer PMH. Mineral trioxide aggregate and other bioactive endodontic cements: an updated overview - Part I: vital pulp therapy. Int Endod J. 2018;51:177. https://doi.org/10.1111/iej.12841.
4. Ha W, Kahler B, Walsh LJ. Classification and nomenclature of commercial hygroscopic dental cements. Eur Endod J. 2017;2:27.
5. Khalil I, Naaman A, Camilleri J. Properties of tricalcium silicate sealers. J Endod. 2016;42:1529–35.
6. Silva Almeida LH, Moraes RR, Morgental RD, Pappen FG. Are premixed calcium silicate–based endodontic sealers comparable to conventional materials? A systematic review of in vitro studies. J Endod. 2017;43:527. https://doi.org/10.1016/j.joen.2016.11.01.
7. Jeong JW, DeGraft-Johnson A, Dorn SO, Di Fiore PM. Dentinal tubule penetration of a calcium silicate–based root canal sealer with different obturation methods. J Endod. 2017;43:633–7.
8. Komabayashi T, Colmenar D, Cvach N, Bhat A, Primus C, Imai Y. Comprehensive review of current endodontic sealers. Dent Mater J. 2020; https://doi.org/10.4012/dmj.2019-288.
9. Primus CM, Tay FR, Niu L-N. Bioactive tri/dicalcium silicate cements for treatment of pulpal and periapical tissues. Acta Biomater. 2019;96:35. https://doi.org/10.1016/j.actbio.2019.05.050.
10. Jiang Y, Zheng Q, Zhou X, Gao Y, Huang D. A comparative study on root canal repair materials: a cytocompatibility assessment in L929 and MG63 cells. ScientificWorldJournal. 2014;2014:463826. https://doi.org/10.1155/2014/463826.
11. Zamparini F, Siboni F, Prati C, Taddei P, Gandolfi MG. Properties of calcium silicate-monobasic calcium phosphate materials for endodontics containing tantalum pentoxide and zirconium oxide. Clin Oral Investig. 2019;23:445–57.
12. De-Deus G, Canabarro A, Alves GG, Marins JR, Linhares ABR, Granjeiro JM. Cytocompatibility

of the ready-to-use bioceramic putty repair cement iRoot BP Plus with primary human osteoblasts. Int Endod J. 2012;45:508. https://doi.org/10.1111/j.1365-2591.2011.02003.x.

13. Tran D, He J, Glickman GN, Woodmansey KF. Comparative analysis of calcium silicate-based root filling materials using an open apex model. J Endod. 2016;42:654–8.

14. Lertmalapong P, Jantarat J, Srisatjaluk RL, Komoltri C. Bacterial leakage and marginal adaptation of various bioceramics as apical plug in open apex model. J Investig Clin Dent. 2019;10:e12371. https://doi.org/10.1111/jicd.12371.

15. Debelian G, Trope M. The use of premixed bioceramic materials in endodontics. G Ital Endod. 2016;30:70. https://doi.org/10.1016/j.gien.2016.09.001.

16. Wang Z. Bioceramic materials in endodontics. Endod Top. 2015;32:3–30.

17. Ree M, Schwartz R. Clinical applications of premixed bioceramic materials in endodontics. Endod Pract. 2015;9:111–27.

18. Xu HHK, Carey LE, Simon CG, Takagi S, Chow LC. Premixed calcium phosphate cements: synthesis, physical properties, and cell cytotoxicity. Dent Mater. 2007;23:433–41.

19. Boyadzhieva E, Dimitrova S, Filipov I, Zagorchev P. Setting time and solubility of premixed bioceramic root canal sealer when applicated with warm gutta percha obturation techniques. IOSR J Dent Med Sci. 2017;16:125–9.

20. Guo Y, Du T, Li H, Shen Y, Mobuchon C, Hieawy A, et al. Physical properties and hydration behavior of a fast-setting bioceramic endodontic material. BMC Oral Health. 2016;16:23. https://doi.org/10.1186/s12903-016-0184-1.

21. Abu Zeid ST, Alamoudi RA, Abou Neel EA, Mokeem Saleh AA. Morphological and spectroscopic study of an apatite layer induced by fast-set versus regular-set EndoSequence root repair materials. Materials (Basel). 2019;12:3678. https://doi.org/10.3390/ma12223678.

22. Lagisetti A, Hegde P, Hegde M. Evaluation of bioceramics and zirconia-reinforced glass ionomer cement in repair of furcation perforations: an in vitro study. J Conserv Dent. 2018;21:184. https://doi.org/10.4103/JCD.JCD_397_16.

23. Luo T, Liu J, Sun Y, Shen Y, Zou L. Cytocompatibility of Biodentine and iRoot FS with human periodontal ligament cells: an *in vitro* study. Int Endod J. 2018;51:779. https://doi.org/10.1111/iej.12889.

24. Tian J, Zhang Y, Lai Z, Li M, Huang Y, Jiang H, et al. Ion release, microstructural, and biological properties of iRoot BP Plus and ProRoot MTA exposed to an acidic environment. J Endod. 2017;43:163–8.

25. Reszka P, Nowicka A, Lipski M, Dura W, Droździk A, Woźniak K. A Comparative chemical study of calcium silicate-containing and epoxy resin-based root canal sealers. Biomed Res Int. 2016;2016:9808432. https://doi.org/10.1155/2016/9808432.

26. Olcay K, Taşli PN, Güven EP, Ülker GMY, Öğüt EE, Çiftçioğlu E, et al. Effect of a novel bioceramic root canal sealer on the angiogenesis-enhancing potential of assorted human odontogenic stem cells compared with principal tricalcium silicate-based cements. J Appl Oral Sci. 2020;28:e20190215. https://doi.org/10.1590/1678-7757-2019-0215.

27. Tibau AV, Grube BD, Velez BJ, Vega VM, Mutter J. Titanium exposure and human health. Oral Sci Int. 2019;16:15. https://doi.org/10.1002/osi2.1001.

28. Camilleri J. Biodentine™ The dentine in a capsule or more? https://www.septodontcorp.com/wp-content/uploads/2018/02/Biodentine-Article-0118-LOW.pdf. Accessed 31 May 2020.

29. Grech L, Mallia B, Camilleri J. Investigation of the physical properties of tricalcium silicate cement-based root-end filling materials. Dent Mater. 2013;29:e20. https://doi.org/10.1016/j.dental.2012.11.007.

30. https://www.septodontcorp.com/files/pdf/ABS-Technology-Brochure.pdf. Accessed 31 May 2020.

31. https://www.septodontusa.com/products/biodentine. Accessed 31 May 2020.

32. Camilleri J, Kralj P, Veber M, Sinagra E. Characterization and analyses of acid-extractable and leached trace elements in dental cements. Int Endod J. 2012;45:737. https://doi.org/10.1111/j.1365-2591.2012.02027.x.

33. Simon S, Flouriot A-C. BioRoot™ RCS a new biomaterial for root canal filling. https://www.septodontusa.com/sites/default/files/2019-04/CSC13_BioRoot%E2%84%A2%20RCS%20a%20new%20biomaterial%20for%20root%20canal%20filling_14.pdf. Accessed 31 May 2020.

34. Asgary S, Shahabi S, Jafarzadeh T, Amini S, Kheirieh S. The properties of a new endodontic material. J Endod. 2008;34:990–3.

35. Kogan P, He J, Glickman GN, Watanabe I. The effects of various additives on setting properties of MTA. J Endod. 2006;32:569–72.

36. Wiltbank KB, Schwartz SA, Schindler WG. Effect of selected accelerants on the physical properties of mineral trioxide aggregate and Portland cement. J Endod. 2007;33:1235–8.

37. Camilleri J, Montesin FE, Papaioannou S, McDonald F, Pitt Ford TR. Biocompatibility of two commercial forms of mineral trioxide aggregate. Int Endod J. 2004;37:699–704.

38. Tanomaru-Filho M, Jorge EG, Guerreiro Tanomaru JM, Gonçalves M. Radiopacity evaluation of new root canal filling materials by digitalization of images. J Endod. 2007;33:249–51.

39. Fonzar F, Mollo A, Venturi M, Pini P, Fonzar RF, Trullenque-Eriksso A, Esposito M. Single versus two visits with 1-week intracanal calcium hydroxide medication for endodontic treatment: one-year post-treatment results from a multicentre randomised controlled trial. Eur J Oral Implantol. 2017;1:29–41.

40. Mehta S, Verma P, Tikku AP, Chandra A, Bains R, Banerjee G. Comparative evaluation of antimicrobial

efficacy of triple antibiotic paste, calcium hydroxide, and a proton pump inhibitor against resistant root canal pathogens. Eur J Dent. 2017;11:53–7.

41. Kvist T, Molander A, Dahlén G, Reit C. Microbiological evaluation of one- and two-visit endodontic treatment of teeth with apical periodontitis: a randomized, clinical trial. J Endod. 2004;30:572–6.

42. Chávez De Paz LE, Dahlén G, Molander A, Möller Å, Bergenholtz G. Bacteria recovered from teeth with apical periodontitis after antimicrobial endodontic treatment. Int Endod J. 2003;36:500–8.

43. http://www.angelusdental.com/img/arquivos/2833_10502833_0111022019_bio_c_temp_bula_fechado.pdf. Accessed 31 May 2020.

44. Guerrero F, Mendoza A, Ribas D, Aspiazu K. Apexification: a systematic review. J Conserv Dent. 2018;21:462. https://doi.org/10.4103/JCD.JCD_96_18.

45. Gharechahi M, Ghoddusi J. A nonsurgical endodontic treatment in open-apex and immature teeth affected by dens invaginatus: using a collagen membrane as an apical barrier. J Am Dent Assoc. 2012;143:144–8.

46. Andreasen JO, Munksgaard EC, Bakland LK. Comparison of fracture resistance in root canals of immature sheep teeth after filling with calcium hydroxide or MTA. Dent Traumatol. 2006;22:154–6.

47. Nosrat A, Nekoofar MH, Bolhari B, Dummer PMH. Unintentional extrusion of mineral trioxide aggregate: a report of three cases. Int Endod J. 2012;45:1165–76.

48. Lin JC, Lu JX, Zeng Q, Zhao W, Li WQ, Ling JQ. Comparison of mineral trioxide aggregate and calcium hydroxide for apexification of immature permanent teeth: a systematic review and meta-analysis. J Formos Med Assoc. 2016;115:523–30.

49. Bücher K, Meier F, Diegritz C, Kaaden C, Hickel R, Kühnisch J. Long-term outcome of MTA apexification in teeth with open apices. Quintessence Int. 2016;47:473. https://doi.org/10.3290/j.qi.a35702.

50. Songtrakul K, Azarpajouh T, Malek M, Sigurdsson A, Kahler B, Lin LM. Modified apexification procedure for immature permanent teeth with a necrotic pulp/apical periodontitis: a case series. J Endod. 2020;46:116–23.

51. Cechella B, de Almeida J, Kuntze M, Felippe W. Analysis of sealing ability of endodontic cements apical plugs. J Clin Exp Dent. 2018;10:146–50.

52. Mente J, Hage N, Pfefferle T, Koch MJ, Dreyhaupt J, Staehle HJ, et al. Mineral trioxide aggregate apical plugs in teeth with open apical foramina: a retrospective analysis of treatment outcome. J Endod. 2009;35:1354–8.

53. Rajasekharan S, Martens LC, Cauwels RGEC, Anthonappa RP. Biodentine™ material characteristics and clinical applications: a 3-year literature review and update. Eur Arch Paediatr Dent. 2018;19:1. https://doi.org/10.1007/s40368-018-0328-x.

54. Martens L, Rajasekharan S, Cauwels R. Endodontic treatment of trauma-induced necrotic immature teeth using a tricalcium silicate-based bioactive cement. A report of 3 cases with 24-month follow-up. Eur J Paediatr Dent. 2016;17:24–8.

55. Sharma S, Sharma V, Passi D, Srivastava D, Grover S, Dutta SR. Large periapical or cystic lesions in association with roots having open apices managed nonsurgically using 1-step apexification based on platelet-rich fibrin matrix and biodentine apical barrier: a case series. J Endod. 2018;44:179–85.

56. Lee LW, Hsiao SH, Lin YH, Chen PY, Lee YL, Hung WC. Outcomes of necrotic immature open-apex central incisors treated by MTA apexification using poly(ε-caprolactone) fiber mesh as an apical barrier. J Formos Med Assoc. 2019;118:362–70.

57. Sisli SN, Ozbas H. Comparative micro–computed tomographic evaluation of the sealing quality of ProRoot MTA and MTA angelus apical plugs placed with various techniques. J Endod. 2017;43:147–51.

58. Drukteinis S, Peciuliene V, Shemesh H, Tusas P, Bendinskaite R. Porosity distribution in apically perforated curved root canals filled with two different calcium silicate-based materials and techniques: a micro-computed tomography study. Materials (Basel). 2019;12:1729. https://doi.org/10.3390/ma12111729.

59. Raveendran DK, Vanamala N, Murali Rao H, Keshava Prasad B, Mankar S, Graduate Student P, et al. Management of open apices with mineral trioxide aggregate and biodentine-a case report. IOSR J Dent Med Sci. 2019;18:9–13.

60. Ng YL, Mann V, Gulabivala K. Outcome of secondary root canal treatment: a systematic review of the literature. Int Endod J. 2008;41:1026. https://doi.org/10.1111/j.1365-2591.2008.01484.x.

61. Mente J, Leo M, Panagidis D, Saure D, Pfefferle T. Treatment outcome of mineral trioxide aggregate: repair of root perforations - long-term results. J Endod. 2014;40:790–6.

62. Gorni FG, Andreano A, Ambrogi F, Brambilla E, Gagliani M. Patient and clinical characteristics associated with primary healing of iatrogenic perforations after root canal treatment: results of a long-term Italian study. J Endod. 2016;42:211–5.

63. Yeung P, Liewehr FR, Moon PC. A quantitative comparison of the fill density of MTA produced by two placement techniques. J Endod. 2006;32:456–9.

64. Tsesis I, Fuss Z. Diagnosis and treatment of accidental root perforations. Endod Top. 2006;13:95. https://doi.org/10.1111/j.1601-1546.2006.00213.x.

65. Tsesis I, Rosenberg E, Faivishevsky V, Kfir A, Katz M, Rosen E. Prevalence and associated periodontal status of teeth with root perforation: a retrospective study of 2,002 patients' medical records. J Endod. 2010;36:797–800.

66. Hamama HH, Yiu CK, Burrow MF, Kahler B, Rossifedele G, Kim HH-E, et al. The influence of cervical preflaring on the amount of apically extruded debris

after root canal preparation using different instrumentation systems. J Endod. 2015;41:1–6.

67. Donnermeyer D, Viedenz A, Schäfer E, Bürklein S. Impact of new cross-sectional designs on the shaping ability of rotary NiTi instruments in S-shaped canals. Odontology. 2020;108:174–9.

68. Schäfer E, Dammaschke T. Development and sequelae of canal transportation. Endod Top. 2006;15:75–90.

69. Razcha C, Zacharopoulos A, Anestis D, Mikrogeorgis G, Zacharakis G, Lyroudia K. Micro-computed tomographic evaluation of canal transportation and centering ability of 4 heat-treated nickel-titanium systems. J Endod. 2020;46:675. https://doi.org/10.1016/j.joen.2020.01.020.

70. Mohammed Saed S, Ashley MP. Root perforations: aetiology, management strategies and outcomes. The hole truth. Br Dent J. 2016;220:171. https://doi.org/10.1038/sj.bdj.2016.132.

71. Lanker A, Fathey W, Samar S, Zakir M, Imranulla M, Pasha S. Non-surgical management of iatrogenic lateral root perforation: a case report. Int J Res Med Sci. 2018;6:1804.

72. Patel B. Iatrogenic perforations. In: Patel B, editor. Endod treatment, retreatment, and surgery. Mastering clinical practice. Cham: Springer International Publishing; 2016. p. 279–96.

73. Aidasani G, Mulay S. Management of iatrogenic errors: furcal perforation. J Int Clin Dent Res Organ. 2018;10:42–6.

74. Pace R, Giuliani V, Pagavino G. Mineral trioxide aggregate as repair material for furcal perforation: case series. J Endod. 2008;34:1130–3.

75. Mancino D, Meyer F, Haikel Y. Improved single visit management of old infected iatrogenic root perforations using Biodentine®. G Ital Endod. 2018;32:17–24.

76. Tek V, Türker SA. A micro-computed tomography evaluation of voids using calcium silicate-based materials in teeth with simulated internal root resorption. Restor Dent Endod. 2019;45:e5. https://doi.org/10.5395/rde.2020.45.e5.

77. Young GR. Contemporary management of lateral root perforation diagnosed with the aid of dental computed tomography. Aust Endod J. 2007;33:112–8.

78. Estrela C, Decurcio DA, Rossi-Fedele G, Silva JA, Guedes OA, Borges ÁH. Root perforations: a review of diagnosis, prognosis and materials. Braz Oral Res. 2018;32:e73. https://doi.org/10.1590/1807-3107bor-2018.vol32.0073.

79. Ha WN, Duckmanton P, Kahler B, Walsh LJ. A survey of various endodontic procedures related to mineral trioxide aggregate usage by members of the Australian Society of Endodontology. Aust Endod J. 2016;42:132–8.

80. Chin JS, Thomas MB, Locke M, Dummer PMH. A survey of dental practitioners in Wales to evaluate the management of deep carious lesions with vital pulp therapy in permanent teeth. Br Dent J. 2016;221:331–8.

81. Guivarc'h M, Jeanneau C, Giraud T, Pommel L, About I, Azim AA, et al. An international survey on the use of calcium silicate-based sealers in non-surgical endodontic treatment. Clin Oral Investig. 2020;24:417–24.

82. https://www.septodont.com.ru/sites/ru/files/2019-07/Septodont_BioRoot_Endo%20sealer%20or%20biological%20filler_JC.pdf. Accessed 31 May 2020.

83. Koch K, Brave DNA. A review of bioceramic technology in endodontics. Roots. 2013;1:6–13.

84. Prati C, Gandolfi MG. Calcium silicate bioactive cements: biological perspectives and clinical applications. Dent Mater. 2015;31:351. https://doi.org/10.1016/j.dental.2015.01.004.

85. Patel S, Ford TP. Is the resorption external or internal? Dent Update. 2007;34:218. https://doi.org/10.12968/denu.2007.34.4.218.

86. Patel S, Ricucci D, Durak C, Tay F. Internal root resorption: a review. J Endod. 2010;36:1107. https://doi.org/10.1016/j.joen.2010.03.014.

87. Roscoe MG, Meira JBC, Cattaneo PM. Association of orthodontic force system and root resorption: a systematic review. Am J Orthod Dentofac Orthop. 2015;147:610. https://doi.org/10.1016/j.ajodo.2014.12.026.

88. Velloso G, de Freitas M, Alves A, Silva A, Barboza E, Moraschini V. Multiple external cervical root resorptions after home whitening treatment: a case report. Aust Dent J. 2017;62:528–33.

89. Fuss Z, Tsesis I, Lin S. Root resorption - diagnosis, classification and treatment choices based on stimulation factors. Dent Traumatol. 2003;19:175–82.

90. Tronstad L. Root resorption - etiology, terminology and clinical manifestations. Dent Traumatol. 1988;4:241–52.

91. Aggarwal V, Singla M. Management of inflammatory root resorption using MTA obturation- a four year follow up. Br Dent J. 2010;208:287–9.

92. Pruthi PJ, Dharmani U, Roongta R, Talwar S. Management of external perforating root resorption by intentional replantation followed by Biodentine restoration. Dent Res J. 2015;12:488–93.

93. Alqedairi A. Non-invasive management of invasive cervical resorption associated with periodontal pocket: a case report. World J Clin Cases. 2019;7:863–71.

94. Mackeviciute M, Subaciene L, Baseviciene N, Siudikiene J. External root resorption - try to save or extract: a case report. J Cont Med A Dent. 2018;3:32–5.

95. Estrela C, Guedes OA, Rabelo LEG, Decurcio DA, Alencar AHG, Estrela CRA, et al. Detection of apical inflammatory root Resorption associated with Periapical lesion using different methods. Braz Dent J. 2014;25:404–8.

96. Laux M, Abbott PV, Pajarola G, Nair PNR. Apical inflammatory root resorption: a correlative radiographic and histological assessment. Int Endod J. 2000;33:483–93.

97. Topçuoğlu HS, Düzgün S, Ceyhanlı KT, Aktı A, Pala K, Kesim B. Efficacy of different irrigation techniques in the removal of calcium hydroxide from a simulated internal root resorption cavity. Int Endod J. 2015;48:309–16.

98. Torres CP, Apicella MJ, Yancich PP, Parker MH. Intracanal placement of calcium hydroxide: a comparison of techniques, revisited. J Endod. 2004;30:225–7.

99. van der Sluis LWM, Wu MK, Wesselink PR. The evaluation of removal of calcium hydroxide paste from an artificial standardized groove in the apical root canal using different irrigation methodologies. Int Endod J. 2007;40:52–7.

100. Nandini S, Velmurugan N, Kandaswamy D. Removal efficiency of calcium hydroxide intracanal medicament with two calcium chelators: volumetric analysis using spiral CT, an in vitro study. J Endod. 2006;32:1097–101.

101. Salzano S, Tirone F. Conservative nonsurgical treatment of class 4 invasive cervical resorption: a case series. J Endod. 2015;41:1907–12.

102. Eftekhar L, Ashraf H, Jabbari S. Management of invasive cervical root resorption in a mandibular canine using biodentine as a restorative material: a case report. Iran Endod J. 2017;12:386–9.

103. Chércoles-Ruiz A, Sánchez-Torres A, Gay-Escoda C. Endodontics, endodontic retreatment, and apical surgery versus tooth extraction and implant placement: a systematic review. J Endod. 2017;43:679. https://doi.org/10.1016/j.joen.2017.01.004.

104. Esposito M, Trullenque-Eriksson A, Tallarico M. Endodontic retreatment versus dental implants of teeth with an uncertain endodontic prognosis: 3-year results from a randomised controlled trial. Eur J Oral Implantol. 2018;11:423–38.

105. Tang Y, Li X, Yin S. Outcomes of MTA as root-end filling in endodontic surgery: a systematic review. Quintessence Int. 2010;41:557–66.

106. Solanki N, Venkappa K, Shah N. Biocompatibility and sealing ability of mineral trioxide aggregate and biodentine as root-end filling material: a systematic review. J Conserv Dent. 2018;21:10. https://doi.org/10.4103/JCD.JCD_45_17.

107. Chen I, Karabucak B, Wang C, Wang HG, Koyama E, Kohli MR, et al. Healing after root-end microsurgery by using mineral trioxide aggregate and a new calcium silicate-based bioceramic material as root-end filling materials in dogs. J Endod. 2015;41:389–99.

108. Tang JJ, Shen ZS, Qin W, Lin Z. A comparison of the sealing abilities between Biodentine and MTA as root-end filling materials and their effects on bone healing in dogs after periradicular surgery. J Appl Oral Sci. 2019;27:e20180693. https://doi.org/10.1590/1678-7757-2018-0693.

109. Vivan RR, Guerreiro-Tanomaru JM, Bernardes RA, Reis JMSN, Hungaro Duarte MA, Tanomaru-Filho M. Effect of ultrasonic tip and root-end filling material on bond strength. Clin Oral Investig. 2016;20:2007–11.

110. Tawil PZ. Periapical microsurgery: can ultrasonic root-end preparations clinically create or propagate dentinal defects? J Endod. 2016;42:1472–5.

111. Floratos S, Kim S. Modern endodontic microsurgery concepts: a clinical update. Dent Clin N Am. 2017;61:81. https://doi.org/10.1016/j.cden.2016.08.007.

Bioceramic Materials in Pediatric Dentistry

Luc C. Martens and Sivaprakash Rajasekharan

1 Introduction

The American Dental Association (ADA) defines pediatric dentistry as "an age-defined specialty that provides both primary and comprehensive preventive and therapeutic oral health care for infants and children through adolescence, including those with special health care needs" and Endodontics as "the branch of dentistry which is concerned with the morphology, physiology and pathology of the human dental pulp and periradicular tissues. Its study and practice encompass the basic and clinical sciences including biology of the normal pulp, the etiology, diagnosis, prevention and treatment of diseases and injuries of the pulp and associated periradicular conditions." By a combination of these definitions, this chapter will cover all endodontic treatment procedures within the age-defined pediatric population.

For decades, the management of the dental pulp in the primary dentition was performed worldwide with semi-toxic products such as Buckley's formocresol and in some countries with iodoform pastes. The latter was especially advocated because of their antibacterial activity and their ability to resorb [1]. With the introduc-

tion of mineral trioxide aggregate (MTA) and, more recently, several new hydraulic tricalcium silicate–based cements, the management of pulpotomy of primary molars has been undertaken using these materials. Furthermore, a more biological treatment approach in deep carious lesions of immature permanent molars became accepted. This change involved a shift of the traditional paradigm regarding excavating all carious dentin with the risk of pulp exposure into the more conservative (i.e., biological) way leaving a thin layer of infected dentin in the cavity and covering this layer with a hydraulic tricalcium silicate–based material. A comparable paradigm shift also exits for the management of traumatized immature permanent incisors with pulpal involvement. After decades of using calcium hydroxide for indirect and direct cappings, pulpotomy, and apexification/apexogenesis procedures, hydraulic tricalcium silicate–based cements have replaced it and are now the materials of choice for all the aforementioned indications owing to its increased desirable interaction with biological tissues.

For the both abovementioned clinical situations—deep carious lesions in the primary molars or the permanent immature molars and in addition after traumatic injuries, calcium silicate–based materials gained enormous attention and use. These cements are hydraulic and a number of them are self-setting materials whose physicochemical properties are suitable for pulp therapy.

L. C. Martens (✉) · S. Rajasekharan
Department of Paediatric Dentistry, School of Oral Health Sciences, Ghent University, Ghent, Belgium
e-mail: luc.martens@ugent.be; Sivaprakash.Rajasekharan@ugent.be

© Springer Nature Switzerland AG 2021
S. Drukteinis, J. Camilleri (eds.), *Bioceramic Materials in Clinical Endodontics*,
https://doi.org/10.1007/978-3-030-58170-1_7

2 Endodontic Management of the Primary Molars

The dental pulp in the primary dentition is histologically similar to that of permanent dentition. Endodontics in the primary dentition is part of the overall treatment plan in young children, especially in the high caries/trauma-risk group. This therapy depends on an accurate diagnosis of the pulp status, and whether the pulp is vital, inflamed or necrotic. It is well known that in 80% of primary teeth with carious exposures, the clinical and radiographic pathology show inflammation that is only limited to the coronal part of the pulp. This is mainly known as *chronic coronal pulpitis*. The different pulpal conditions in the primary teeth are summarized in Table 1 [2]:

Knowledge on pulp response to caries and being able to interpret symptoms correctly is of utmost importance whether performing a rather conservative treatment (stepwise excavation, indirect pulp capping), an intermediate invasive treatment (direct pulp capping), or a radical intervention (partial and full pulpotomy) (Table 2 and Fig. 1).

The following factors should be considered during the decision-making for an endodontic intervention.

Table 1 Differentiation of clinical conditions and pulpal consequences in primary teeth

Clinical condition	Pulpal consequences
Healthy pulp	When exposed due to trauma or accidentally during cavity preparation. The pulp can be kept healthy if properly treated.
Deep carious lesions	Can cause inflammation of the pulp before the pulp is exposed. This is especially the case with proximal exposures. This condition can be reversible or irreversible depending on patient's symptoms and extensive bleeding during therapy.
Carious exposed pulp	Are always inflamed partially or totally, or may be necrotic.
Partial or total pulpal necrosis	May be the consequence of untreated caries or traumatically exposed pulp.

Table 2 Endodontic techniques[a] for primary teeth (after Duggal and Nazzal [2])

Therapy	Procedures	Indications
Stepwise excavation	Removal of most carious dentin. Demineralized dentin covered with glass-ionomer lining and cement and left temporarily under an intermediate restoration	Deep carious lesion, carious softened tissue close to pulp but no exposure. No clinical signs of pulpitis
Indirect pulp capping	Removal of almost all the carious dentin. Affected dentin covered with glass-ionomer lining	Deep carious lesion, carious softened tissue close to pulp but no exposure. No clinical or some radiographic signs of pulpitis
Direct pulp capping	No surgical removal of exposed pulp tissue. Pulp covered with a bioceramic material	Accidental minimal exposure of healthy pulp during preparation or via trauma. Little or no contamination of the exposed area
Partial pulpotomy	Excision of a superficial part of the pulp. A bioceramic material should be applied in tissue contact with the wound without an extra pulpal blood clot	Accidental exposure of healthy pulp; carious exposure-partial chronic pulpitis
Pulpotomy	Removal of the coronal pulp. Wound surfaces placed in the orifices of the root canals	Carious exposure—pulpitis, partial or coronal chronic pulpitis, marginal ridge breakdown

[a]Pulpectomy was not included in the table because this technique should have a very limited use. From a clinical point of view, it can be considered if there is an irreversible pulpitis including the entire pulp system or in the presence of necrotic pulp or acute infection. However, there are a lot of considerations necessary for making this decision (see below). In a case where the second premolar is missing, while the retention of the primary molar is required for orthodontic reasons, pulpectomy can maybe be considered [2]

Fig. 1 Schematic representation of endodontic therapies in primary molars. (Drawings used with permission of Wiley-Blackwell)

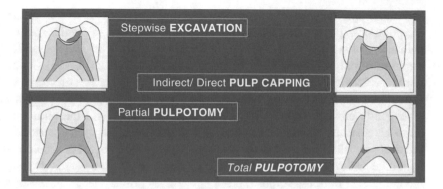

- Pulpal diagnosis
- Occlusal considerations
- The patient's ability to cooperate. Can the treatment be performed conventionally or is sedation/general anesthesia needed?
- Patient's general and oral health
- Patient's and parent's motivation and consent
- Patient's caries risk
- The risk of injury/infection of the underlying permanent tooth germ
- The effect of the proposed endodontic intervention on the patient's health, for example, infective endocarditis in children who have congenital heart defects or have had heart surgery
- The effect of the proposed endodontic intervention on the underlying permanent tooth germ

All these factors should help the clinician in his decision whether to keep or extract the tooth [2].

2.1 Stepwise Excavation and Indirect Pulp Capping

During stepwise excavation, the soft part of carious dentine is removed and dentine floor is covered with a glass-ionomer liner and the tooth is completely filled with a semi-permanent filling material. Secondary dentin formation during at least 3–6 months will lead to less risk of exposing the pulp during further excavation of carious dentin [3, 4]. This technique, however, is not recommended as a favored approach for deep carious

lesions in primary molars for children because another appointment with the administration of local anesthesia should be avoided. In cases where reversible pulpitis is diagnosed, a single-visit indirect capping must be considered. During this procedure, removal of almost all carious dentin is performed and affected dentin will be covered with hydraulic tricalcium silicate–based cements, and the tooth will be permanently restored.

2.2 Direct Pulp Capping

Direct pulp capping is well known as a technique whereby the exposed vital pulp is capped with a medicament. For many years, this was preferably performed using calcium hydroxide. It has been shown that inflammation of the pulp precedes the exposure of the pulp [5, 6]. Dentinal tubules are wide in primary molars, and bacteria penetrate the pulp, causing inflammation before clinically being exposed. For that reason, direct capping should not be considered if the exposure resulted from caries excavation. The only situation where direct pulp capping could be considered in primary teeth is where pulp exposure is traumatic and not due to the caries [7]. Nowadays, hydraulic tricalcium silicate–based cements are recommended for these purposes [8, 9].

2.3 Partial Pulpotomy

In cases of healthy pulp exposure or partial chronic pulpitis, a partial pulpotomy is the treatment of choice. However, the clinician should be sure that pupal inflammation is very localized at the point of exposure. Any history of continuous pain after cold or heat or continuous pain indicating signs of pulpitis should be excluded, and only normal bleeding after pulpotomy procedure should be seen. This bleeding must be controlled after gentle pressure with a wet cotton pellet. If more hemostasis is needed, the clinician should proceed to the full pulpotomy. Nowadays, hydraulic tricalcium silicate based–cements are recommended for these purposes [10, 11].

2.4 Pulpotomy, Wound Dressing, Tissue Reaction, and Outcome

The most widely used vital pulp therapy technique for the treatment of deciduous teeth with carious pulp exposure is pulpotomy. According to the American Academy of Pediatric Dentistry, a pulpotomy is defined as the ablation of infected or affected pulp tissues leaving the residual vital pulp tissues intact, thus preserving vitality and function (totally or partially) of the radicular pulp, while the remaining pulp stump is covered with a medicament [12]. The rationale for pulpotomy is based on the assumption that inflammation and impaired vascularity caused by the bacterial invasion is confined to the superficial part of the coronal pulp, while the radicular pulp tissue remains functional. The primary objective in the treatment of the tooth with pulpal involvement is to retain it in a functional state (mastication, phonation, swallowing, and esthetics), so that it may fulfil its role as a useful component of the primary and young permanent dentition [13].

Pulpectomy should be avoided because of the risk of infecting the underlying permanent tooth germ, the number of accessory canals which can be assessed, and the difficulty to find a resorbable material [14]. As stated above, there is limited indication and if so, the use of hydraulic tricalcium silicate based–cements will not be an option as they are not resorbable [15].

An ideal pulpotomy agent must be bactericidal, promote healing of the radicular pulp, be biocompatible, offer the dentine–pulp complex a relatively stable environment, support the regeneration of dentine–pulp complex, and not interfere with the physiological process of root resorption [13, 16]. Covering the floor of the pulp chamber is crucial, in order to ensure that the auxiliary canals traversing to the furcation are sealed and the pulp can thus benefit from the effect of applied materials.

For decades, calcium hydroxide was used as a biological wound dressing on the dental pulp. In primary teeth, however, clinical outcomes were poor with the most cited failure reported as internal resorption [17]. This can be explained by the fact that in most cases where pulp therapy is required, the pulp is chronically inflamed, and calcium hydroxide has no healing effect inflamed pulp. It thus should no longer be used on primary pulp tissue.

Although not biologic, leakage of drug and leaving the pulp in a metastable condition having no healing effect, formocresol (well known as Buckley's formocresol) was worldwide used for many years. The success rate can be estimated between 50% and 95%. Since the International Agency for Research on Cancer classified formaldehyde as a carcinogenic to humans [18], efforts have been made to ban formocresol in endodontic therapy.

Iodoform-based pastes were developed as an alternative to formocresol and have a long-term bactericidal effect. Compared to formocresol, there was no diffusion into the inter- and periradicular area and so less or no toxicity. Success rates were 87–95% [19]. A combination of a fast-setting calcium hydroxide–iodoform-silicone paste showed 100% clinical success and 97% radiographical success [20].

In the last decade, regeneration approaches include pulpotomy agents that have the cell-inductive capacity to either replace lost cells or induce existing cells to differentiate into hard tissue–forming elements. However, iodoform-based pastes did not induce tissue regeneration and were not bioinductive. As a consequence, the trend nowadays is towards the use of bioactive materials to promote the healing of the pulp and keeping the teeth in the dentition. Since the availability of hydraulic tricalcium silicate–based cements and the great clinical success in endodontic therapy, formocresol has been replaced by hydraulic tricalcium silicate–based cements.

From a comparison of MTA (ProRoot Dentsply) and formocresol in 60 pulpotomies randomly selected in 46, 7-year olds, MTA was shown to be a valuable and safe alternative. After 24 months, there was no difference in clinical and radiographic success [21]. The same was shown for a comparison of formocresol with MTA (Angelus) in 45 pulpotomies in 23 children (5–9 years). In the MTA group, dentin bridges were seen in 29% of cases [22]. From a limited systematic review [23], it was suggested that the use of MTA is the best clinical practice. Regardless of the limited evidence [24], the use of MTA became generally accepted for vital pulpotomy in primary molars. Figure 2 illustrates a number of studies with the clinical outcome for formocresol versus MTA [22, 25–33]. From this figure, it can be concluded that on average the clinical outcome of MTA at least equals or is slightly better compared to formocresol.

Besides MTA, other hydraulic tricalcium silicate based–cements can be considered for pulpotomy in the primary dentition. Although, several cements are referred to as hydraulic tricalcium silicate–based cements, they can be classified based on their origin of tricalcium silicate as either Portland cement derivatives (MTA and its formulations) or laboratory synthesized (Biodentine™, BioAggregate, EndoSequence, and iRoot BP). The laboratory-synthesized hydraulic tricalcium silicate–based materials have different characteristics to the original formulation of MTA; this includes elimination of aluminum, addition of alternative radiopacifiers, minimizing particle size, and additives to enhance physical properties. Biodentine™ incorporates all of these changes in the cement composition and its clinical efficiency in pulp therapy has been compared with MTA in the following sections.

Biodentine™ is a hydraulic tricalcium silicate–based inorganic nonmetallic restorative cement commercialized and advertised as a "bioactive dentine substitute" [34]. The material is claimed to possess far better physical and biological properties such as material handling [35], faster setting time [36], increased compressive strength [37], increased density [38], decreased

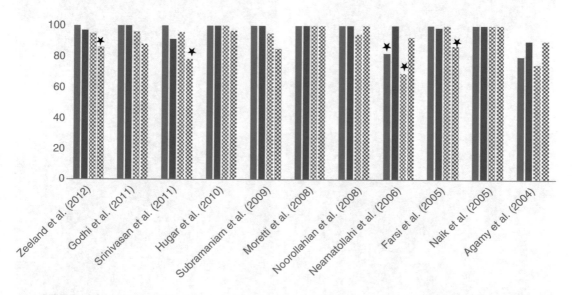

■ MTA clincial outcome   ■ FC clinical outcome   ✾ MTA radiographic outcome   ✾ FC radiographic outcome

Fig. 2 An overview of clinical and radiographic success rate comparison between formocresol and MTA in primary molar pulpotomies. The asterisk indicates significant difference between the outcomes

porosity [39], and induction of reparative dentine synthesis [40] when compared to similar material types [41, 42].

The very first randomized clinical trial (RCT) on Biodentine™ in primary molar pulpotomy was a parallel-design RCT comparing it to ProRoot White MTA [43]. Patients above 3 years of age with carious primary teeth with vital pulps without spontaneous pain or history of swelling were included. Fifty-eight patients (82 teeth) with a mean age of 4.79 ± 1.23 years were included. The teeth were randomized, blinded, and allocated to one of the three groups (Biodentine™, ProRoot® White MTA (WMTA) or Tempophore™) for pulpotomy treatment. All teeth were followed up clinically and radiographically (after 6, 12, and 18 months) by two-blinded calibrated investigators. Forty-six patients and 69 teeth were available for follow-up after 18 months. Clinical success (radiographic success in parenthesis) was 95.24% (94.4%), 100%

(90.9%), and 95.65% (82.4%) in the Biodentine™, ProRoot® WMTA, and Tempophore™ groups, respectively, but the difference was not significant. Pulp canal obliteration was significantly different amongst the experimental groups as the Biodentine™ group exhibited significantly more pulp canal obliteration when compared to the WMTA group at 6 months ($P = 0.008$) and the 18 months ($P = 0.003$). One of the cases is illustrated in Fig. 3. From this RCT, it could be concluded that after 18-month follow-up, there was no significant difference between Biodentine™ in comparison with White ProRoot MTA or Tempophore™.

In the meantime, several other studies became published comparing MTA with Biodentine™ [43–52]. The clinical success rates vary between 60% and 100% (Fig. 4). However, except for one study [50], the overall clinical success rate of both hydraulic tricalcium silicate–based cements is higher than 90%.

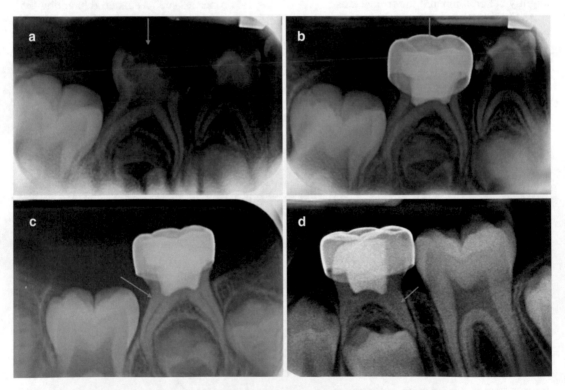

Fig. 3 The Biodentine case series with 18 months follow-up. Arrows indicate the region of interest (a) preoperative radiograph (b) immediate postoperative (c) dentine bridge formation and pulp canal obliteration (d)

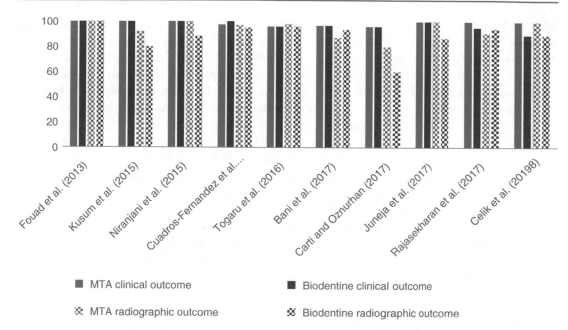

■ MTA clinical outcome ■ Biodentine clinical outcome

� MTA radiographic outcome � Biodentine radiographic outcome

Fig. 4 The clinical and radiographic success rates of various studies comparing MTA and Biodentine™ in primary molar pulpotomy. No significant differences between the two materials were observed

2.5 Clinical Procedure

The following steps should be followed:
- Administration of local anesthesia.
- Application of rubber dam.
- Caries removal and coronal access using a high-speed cylindrical diamond bur with ample water spray.
- Removal of the coronal pulp or with a sterile bur or with a sterile spoon excavator.
- Checking root canal orifices.
- Normal hemostasis by application of light pressure with a wet cotton pellet. Additional tools can be calcium hydroxide powder or cellulose pellets. If hemostasis was not obtained within 5 min [17], pulp tissue in the canal was assumed to be infected, and then extraction should be considered (see above).
- Application of minimum of 2 mm layer of the pulpotomy agent according to the manufacturer's instructions.
- Coverage with appropriate cement is needed in case of ProRoot MTA applications. For Biodentine™, the wound dressing can also fill up the entire pulp chamber and even be used as a temporary filling. The latter is a major

advantage compared to other hydraulic tricalcium silicate–based cements. However, several other hydraulic tricalcium silicate–based cements could also be used for this purpose and the restoration protocol depends on the type of cement used.
- The final restoration can be obtained with adhesive restorations or stainless steel crowns.

In this respect, the clinician should be aware of the fact that healing of the dental pulp is not exclusively dependent on the supposed stimulatory effect of a particular type of agent but is also directly related to the capacity of both the dressing and permanent restorative material to provide a biological seal against immediate and long-term microleakage along the entire restoration interface [53]. Stainless steel crowns protect the underlying pulp against leakage and are a necessity for the long-term success of vital pulp therapy in cariously exposed teeth [54, 55]. The use of stainless steel crowns increases the success rate of pulpotomy. In case there is a choice for MTA and an esthetic filling on top, one should be aware of potential discoloration. Especially, MTAs with bismuth oxide will cause grayish discoloration. MTAs with other radiopacifiers or other hydraulic tricalcium silicate based–cements with alternative radiopacifiers will have no or significantly less discoloration [56].

3 Deep Carious Lesions in Immature First Permanent Molars

In time, deep caries management was performed to "extension for prevention" principles which were destructive with complete removal of all carious dentine. Thanks to the "adhesive" dental materials, minimal invasive dentistry (i.e., prevention of extension) with selective caries removal became accepted worldwide. In the last two decades, with the evolution into hydraulic tricalcium silicate–based cements, biological treatment strategies have been advocated.

From a recent consensus document, deep caries was defined as radiographic evidence of caries reaching the inner third or inner quarter of dentine with a risk of pulp exposure [57]. Clinically, the depth of caries and residual dentine thickness are difficult to assess [58]. Recent research on deep carious tissue management supports less invasive strategies. Most recently, leaving a thin layer of infected dentine covered by these new materials is recommended [57]. With these approaches, reduced risk of pulp exposure and pulp healing are obtained. Management strategies for the treatment of cariously exposed pulp are also shifting with avoidance of pulpectomy and the reemergence of vital pulp treatment techniques such as partial and complete pulpotomy. Especially, the development of MTA and other hydraulic calcium silicates has resulted in more predictable treatments from both a histological and a clinical perspective [59].

This approach is of particular interest in deep carious immature first permanent molars. In these young children, an invasive endodontic treatment can be avoided. Figure 5a–d illustrates a full pulpotomy on a first permanent molar in the third quadrant and an indirect capping on the contralateral molar in a 10-year-old boy. The procedures performed were exactly the same as described earlier for the primary teeth. In both cases, Biodentine™ was used. Although it is perfectly possible to keep this hydraulic calcium silicate–based cement for at least 6 months in the mouth as a provisionary filling [60] having a second visit for permanent restoration, a one-visit treatment is also allowed and recommended. The setting time of Biodentine™ (i.e., up to 12 min according to manufacturer's instructions) is a bit crucial, but a recent report showed that after 3 min one could put permanent adhesive materials on top [61].

4 Pulpotomy in Traumatized Immature Teeth

Crown fractures with pulp exposure represent 18–20% of traumatic injuries involving the teeth, the majority being in young permanent central incisors [62]. These injuries produce changes in the exposed pulp tissues, and a biological and functional restoration of immature young permanent teeth represents an important clinical challenge [63]. The treatment plan in such cases is to maintain pulp vitality via apexogenesis, which allows continued root development along the entire root length [64]. Apexogenesis after traumatic exposure in vital young permanent teeth can be accomplished by implementing the appropriate vital pulp therapy such as pulp capping (direct or indirect) or pulpotomy (partial or complete) depending on the time between the trauma and treatment of the patient, degree of root development, and size of the pulp exposure [65]. Histologic examination of traumatized pulp shows that the depth of inflammatory reaction does not exceed 2 mm from the exposed surface within 48 h [66]. Therefore, if treated within 48 h, 2 mm of the injured pulp can be successfully removed, leaving the non-inflamed healthy radicular pulp to reorganize.

In this era of regenerative endodontics, it is of utmost importance to define the real meaning of regenerative endodontics. As long as the vital pulp is present where we use hydraulic tricalcium silicate–based cements, we are performing a therapy which repairs the dentin–pulp complex. When we are revitalizing teeth using the fresh blood in canals and using hydraulic tricalcium silicate–based cements in combination with/ without scaffolds, we are promoting the regeneration of new (dental) tissue [67]. According to the above, the goal of treating dental trauma in immature incisors is to perform a therapy to repair the dentin–pulp complex. Figure 6 illustrates MTA pulpotomies in two immature maxillary incisors. The procedure is the same as explained in Sect. 2.5.

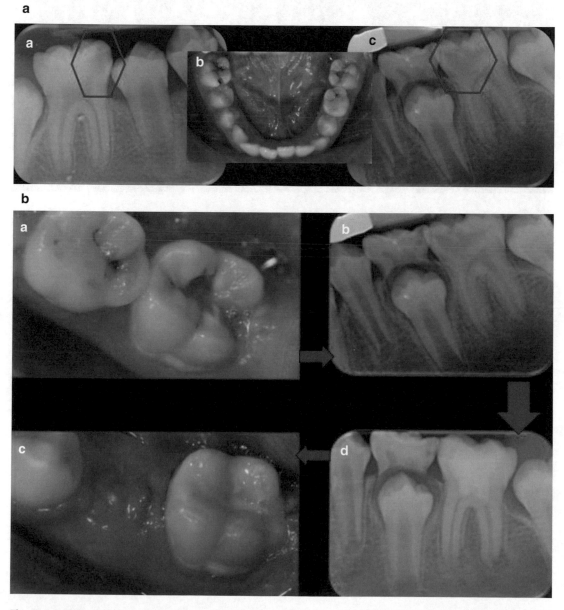

Fig. 5 (**a**) Clinical (b) and radiographical (a, c) illustrations of deep caries in the 4.6 (a) and extremely deep carious in the 3.6 (c) in a 10-year-old boy. (**b**) Clinical and radiographical illustrations of extremely deep carious in the 36 (a, b). A Biodentine™ pulpotomy was performed (c) followed by an imm0ediate adhesive restoration (d). (**c**) Deep carious lesion (a, e); cavity preparation (b); indirect capping with Biodentine™ (c, f) followed by an immediate adhesive restoration (d). (**d**) Radiographical follow-up from baseline up to 18 months (a–f) showing the formation of dentin bridges (c) or extensively hard tissue formation (f) and further apexogenesis (c, f)

c

d

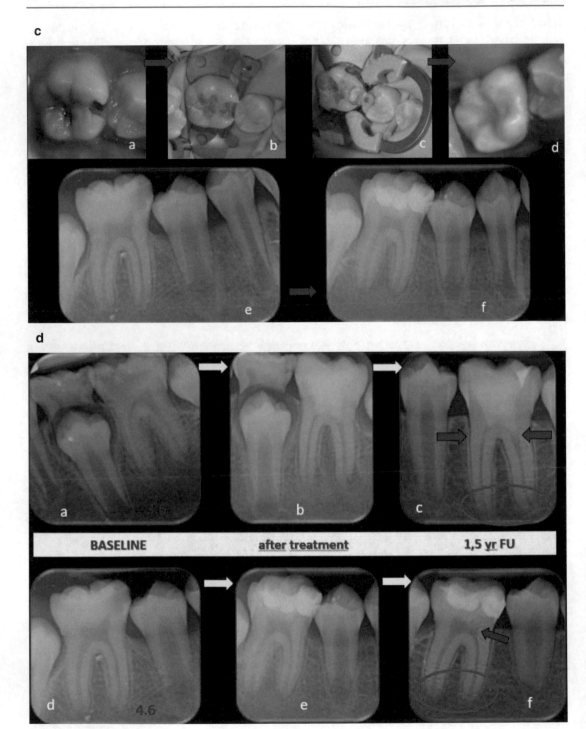

Fig. 5 (continued)

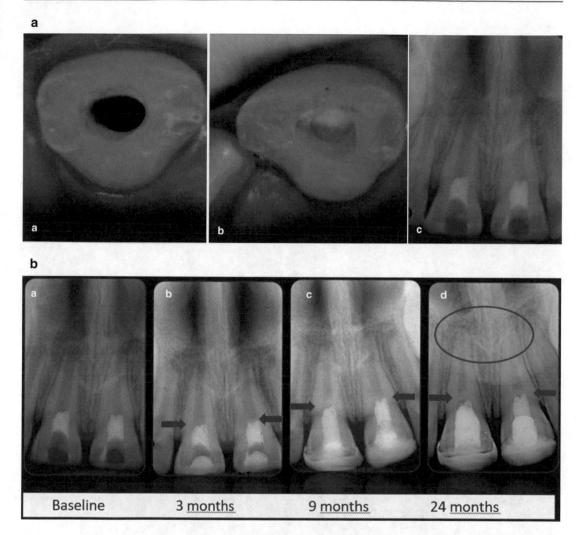

Fig. 6 (**a**) MTA pulpotomies in two central incisors. Teeth were further opened after injury and pulp was removed from the chamber (a), after hemostasis pulp was covered with MTA (b). X-ray control was performed (c). Courtesy to R. Cauwels, Dept Paed Dent, UGent. (**b**) 24 months radiographical follow-up after MTA pulpotomy (a–d) with early signs of dentin bridge formation (b), extending (c) combined with full apexogenesis (c, d). Courtesy to R. Cauwels, Dept Paed Dent, UGent

In another 7-year-old Caucasian female who visited the emergency service after she had an accident in the playground, an enamel dentine fracture with pulp exposure with respect to tooth 11 was diagnosed (Fig. 7a). Due to severe anxiety, treatment under local analgesia was impossible. The treatment was performed the following day under general anesthesia. The pulp exposure was further opened with a sterile high-speed diamond bur with sufficient water cooling. The pulp tissue until the cement–enamel junction was removed (complete pulpotomy). Pulp capping or partial pulpotomy was not a viable option in this instance as the duration of between trauma and treatment was more than 24 h. Hemostasis was achieved with a moist cotton pellet, and the pulp exposure was capped with Biodentine™ and used as a temporary filling. A radiograph at this appointment showed an immature open apex, and the

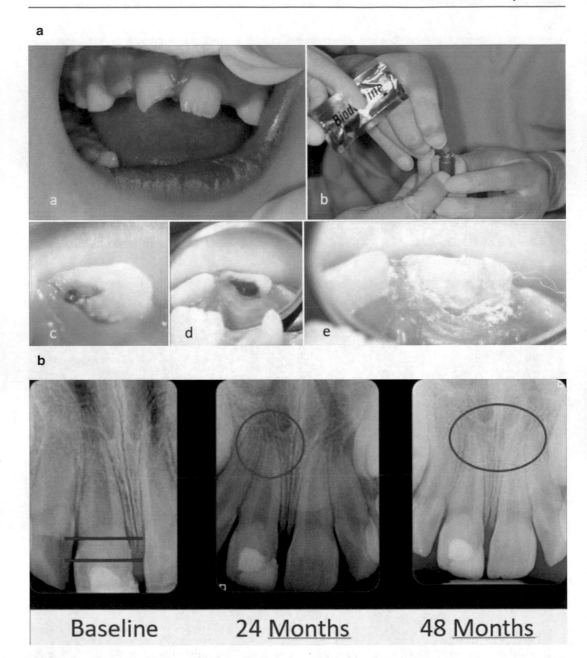

Fig. 7 (**a**) A 7-year-old girl presented with a complex crown fracture with pulp exposure (a, c). After further opening (d) a Biodentine™ pulpotomy was performed (b, e). This bioceramic was also holded as a provisionary filling. (**b**) Radiographical follow-up after Biodentine™ pulpotomy up to 48 months with full apexogenesis

Biodentine™ pulpotomy could be noted at the cingulum level. Three weeks later, a permanent composite restoration was made. Clinical tooth vitality and digital radiographical evaluation were performed after 6, 12, 18, 24, and 48 months (Fig. 7b). No subjective discomfort was reported during the entire follow-up period. Clinically, the tooth remained vital, and no discoloration was observed. Radiographically, starting from 18 months, complete apexogenesis was evident, and this was further confirmed at the 24- and 48-month follow-up.

5 Conclusions

With the better understanding of the dentin–pulp complex and its molecular biology in conjunction with the development of newer materials especially based on hydraulic tricalcium silicate cements, a total paradigm shift has become possible for the management of deep carious lesions in the primary dentition and in immature permanent molars as well as in traumatic injuries. The use of hydraulic tricalcium silicate–based materials in pediatric endodontics is the best clinical practice with a most favorable outcome.

References

1. Cerqueira DF, Mello-Moura AC, Santos EM, Guedes-Pinto AC. Cytotoxicity, histopathological, microbiological and clinical aspects of an endodontic iodoform-based paste used in pediatric dentistry: a review. J Clin Pediatr Dent. 2008;32(2):105–10. https://doi.org/10.17796/jcpd.32.2.k1wx5571 h2w85430.
2. Duggal MS, Nazzal H. Endodontic management of primary teeth. In: Koch G, editor. Pediatric dentistry. London: Wiley Blackwell; 2017.
3. Bjorndal L. Indirect pulp therapy and stepwise excavation. Pediatr Dent. 2008;30(3):225–9.
4. Bjorndal L, Simon S, Tomson PL, Duncan HF. Management of deep caries and the exposed pulp. Int Endod J. 2019;52(7):949–73. https://doi.org/10.1111/iej.13128.
5. Duggal MS, Nooh A, High A. Response of the primary pulp to inflammation: a review of the Leeds studies and challenges for the future. Eur J Paediatr Dent. 2002;3(3):111–4.
6. Kassa D, Day P, High A, Duggal M. Histological comparison of pulpal inflammation in primary teeth with occlusal or proximal caries. Int J Paediatr Dent. 2009;19(1):26–33. https://doi.org/10.1111/j.1365-263X.2008.00962.x.
7. Duggal M, Tong HJ, Al-Ansary M, Twati W, Day PF, Nazzal H. Interventions for the endodontic management of non-vital traumatised immature permanent anterior teeth in children and adolescents: a systematic review of the evidence and guidelines of the European Academy of Paediatric Dentistry. Eur Arch Paediatr Dent. 2017;18(3):139–51. https://doi.org/10.1007/s40368-017-0289-5.
8. Asl Aminabadi N, Satrab S, Najafpour E, Samiei M, Jamali Z, Shirazi S. A randomized trial of direct pulp capping in primary molars using MTA compared to 3Mixtatin: a novel pulp capping biomaterial. Int J Paediatr Dent. 2016;26(4):281–90. https://doi.org/10.1111/ipd.12196.
9. Smail-Faugeron V, Glenny AM, Courson F, Durieux P, Muller-Bolla M, Fron Chabouis H. Pulp treatment for extensive decay in primary teeth. Cochrane Database Syst Rev. 2018;5:CD003220. https://doi.org/10.1002/14651858.CD003220.pub3.
10. Martens L, Rajasekharan S, Cauwels R. Pulp management after traumatic injuries with a tricalcium silicate-based cement (Biodentine): a report of two cases, up to 48 months follow-up. Eur Arch Paediatr Dent. 2015;16(6):491–6. https://doi.org/10.1007/s40368-015-0191-y.
11. Nematollahi H, Noorollahian H, Bagherian A, Yarbakht M, Nematollahi S. Mineral trioxide aggregate partial pulpotomy versus formocresol pulpotomy: a randomized, split-mouth, controlled clinical trial with 24 months follow-up. Pediatr Dent. 2018;40(3):184–9.
12. American Academy on Pediatric Dentistry Clinical Affairs Committee-Pulp Therapy s, American Academy on Pediatric Dentistry Council on Clinical A. Guideline on pulp therapy for primary and young permanent teeth. Pediatr Dent. 2008;30(7 Suppl):170–4.
13. Fuks AB. Pulp therapy for the primary and young permanent dentitions. Dent Clin North Am. 2000;44(3):571–96, vii.
14. Garcia-Godoy F. Evaluation of an iodoform paste in root canal therapy for infected primary teeth. ASDC J Dent Child. 1987;54(1):30–4.
15. Ranly DM, Garcia-Godoy F. Current and potential pulp therapies for primary and young permanent teeth. J Dent. 2000;28(3):153–61. https://doi.org/10.1016/s0300-5712(99)00065-2.
16. Zhang W, Yelick PC. Vital pulp therapy-current progress of dental pulp regeneration and revascularization. Int J Dent. 2010;2010:856087. https://doi.org/10.1155/2010/856087.
17. Vargas KG, Fuks AB, Peretz B. Pulpotomy techniques: cervical (traditional) and partial. In: Paediatric endodontics, current concepts in pulp therapy for primary and young permanent teeth. Berlin: Springer; 2016.
18. Humans IWGotEoCRt. Formaldehyde, 2-butoxyethanol and 1-tert-butoxypropan-2-ol. IARC Monogr Eval Carcinog Risks Hum. 2006;88:1–478.
19. Boeve C, Dermaut L. Formocresol pulpotomy in primary molars: a long-term radiographic evaluation. ASDC J Dent Child. 1982;49(3):191–6.
20. Nurko C, Garcia-Godoy F. Evaluation of a calcium hydroxide/iodoform paste (Vitapex) in root canal therapy for primary teeth. J Clin Pediatr Dent. 1999;23(4):289–94.
21. Noorollahian H. Comparison of mineral trioxide aggregate and formocresol as pulp medicaments for pulpotomies in primary molars. Br Dent J. 2008;204(11):E20. https://doi.org/10.1038/sj.bdj.2008.319.
22. Moretti AB, Sakai VT, Oliveira TM, Fornetti AP, Santos CF, Machado MA, et al. The effectiveness

of mineral trioxide aggregate, calcium hydroxide and formocresol for pulpotomies in primary teeth. Int Endod J. 2008;41(7):547–55. https://doi.org/10.1111/j.1365-2591.2008.01377.x.

23. Simancas-Pallares MA, Diaz-Caballero AJ, Luna-Ricardo LM. Mineral trioxide aggregate in primary teeth pulpotomy. A systematic literature review. Med Oral Patol Oral Cir Bucal. 2010;15(6):e942–6. https://doi.org/10.4317/medoral.15.e942.

24. Anthonappa RP, King NM, Martens LC. Is there sufficient evidence to support the long-term efficacy of mineral trioxide aggregate (MTA) for endodontic therapy in primary teeth? Int Endod J. 2013;46(3):198–204. https://doi.org/10.1111/j.1365-2591.2012.02128.x.

25. Godhi B, Sood PB, Sharma A. Effects of mineral trioxide aggregate and formocresol on vital pulp after pulpotomy of primary molars: an in vivo study. Contemp Clin Dent. 2011;2(4):296–301. https://doi.org/10.4103/0976-237X.91792.

26. Srinivasan D, Jayanthi M. Comparative evaluation of formocresol and mineral trioxide aggregate as pulpotomy agents in deciduous teeth. Indian J Dent Res. 2011;22(3):385–90. https://doi.org/10.4103/0970-9290.87058.

27. Hugar SM, Deshpande SD. Comparative investigation of clinical/radiographical signs of mineral trioxide aggregate and formocresol on pulpotomized primary molars. Contemp Clin Dent. 2010;1(3):146–51. https://doi.org/10.4103/0976-237X.72779.

28. Subramaniam P, Konde S, Mathew S, Sugnani S. Mineral trioxide aggregate as pulp capping agent for primary teeth pulpotomy: 2 year follow up study. J Clin Pediatr Dent. 2009;33(4):311–4. https://doi.org/10.17796/jcpd.33.4.r83r38423x58h38w.

29. Farsi N, Alamoudi N, Balto K, Mushayt A. Success of mineral trioxide aggregate in pulpotomized primary molars. J Clin Pediatr Dent. 2005;29(4):307–11. https://doi.org/10.17796/jcpd.29.4.n80t77w625118k73.

30. Naik S, Hegde AH. Mineral trioxide aggregate as a pulpotomy agent in primary molars: an in vivo study. J Indian Soc Pedod Prev Dent. 2005;23(1):13–6. https://doi.org/10.4103/0970-4388.16020.

31. Agamy HA, Bakry NS, Mounir MM, Avery DR. Comparison of mineral trioxide aggregate and formocresol as pulp-capping agents in pulpotomized primary teeth. Pediatr Dent. 2004;26(4):302–9.

32. Zealand CM, Briskie DM, Botero TM, Boynton JR, Hu JC. Comparing gray mineral trioxide aggregate and diluted formocresol in pulpotomized human primary molars. Pediatr Dent. 2010;32(5):393–9.

33. Neamatollahi H, Tajik A. Comparison of clinical and radiographic success rates of pulpotomy in primary molars using Formocresol, Ferric Sulfate and Mineral Trioxide Aggregate (MTA). J Dent (Tehran). 2006;3:6–14.

34. Zanini M, Sautier JM, Berdal A, Simon S. Biodentine induces immortalized murine pulp cell differentiation into odontoblast-like cells and stimulates biominer-alization. J Endod. 2012;38(9):1220–6. https://doi.org/10.1016/j.joen.2012.04.018.

35. Nowicka A, Lipski M, Parafiniuk M, Sporniak-Tutak K, Lichota D, Kosierkiewicz A, et al. Response of human dental pulp capped with biodentine and mineral trioxide aggregate. J Endod. 2013;39(6):743–7. https://doi.org/10.1016/j.joen.2013.01.005.

36. Kaup M, Schafer E, Dammaschke T. An in vitro study of different material properties of Biodentine compared to ProRoot MTA. Head Face Med. 2015;11:16. https://doi.org/10.1186/s13005-015-0074-9.

37. Elnaghy AM, Elsaka SE. Fracture resistance of simulated immature teeth filled with Biodentine and white mineral trioxide aggregate – an in vitro study. Dent Traumatol. 2016;32(2):116–20. https://doi.org/10.1111/edt.12224.

38. Camilleri J, Grech L, Galea K, Keir D, Fenech M, Formosa L, et al. Porosity and root dentine to material interface assessment of calcium silicate-based root-end filling materials. Clin Oral Investig. 2014;18(5):1437–46. https://doi.org/10.1007/s00784-013-1124-y.

39. Gandolfi MG, Siboni F, Botero T, Bossu M, Riccitiello F, Prati C. Calcium silicate and calcium hydroxide materials for pulp capping: biointeractivity, porosity, solubility and bioactivity of current formulations. J Appl Biomater Funct Mater. 2015;13(1):43–60. https://doi.org/10.5301/jabfm.5000201.

40. Nowicka A, Wilk G, Lipski M, Kolecki J, Buczkowska-Radlinska J. Tomographic evaluation of reparative dentin formation after direct pulp capping with Ca(OH)2, MTA, Biodentine, and dentin bonding system in human teeth. J Endod. 2015;41(8):1234–40. https://doi.org/10.1016/j.joen.2015.03.017.

41. Rajasekharan S, Martens LC, Cauwels RG, Verbeeck RM. Biodentine material characteristics and clinical applications: a review of the literature. Eur Arch Paediatr Dent. 2014;15(3):147–58. https://doi.org/10.1007/s40368-014-0114-3.

42. Rajasekharan S, Martens LC, Cauwels R, Anthonappa RP, Verbeeck RMH. Biodentine material characteristics and clinical applications: a 3 year literature review and update. Eur Arch Paediatr Dent. 2018;19(1):1–22. https://doi.org/10.1007/s40368-018-0328-x.

43. Rajasekharan S, Martens LC, Vandenbulcke J, Jacquet W, Bottenberg P, Cauwels RG. Efficacy of three different pulpotomy agents in primary molars: a randomized control trial. Int Endod J. 2017;50(3):215–28. https://doi.org/10.1111/iej.12619.

44. Stringhini Junior E, Dos Santos MGC, Oliveira LB, Mercade M. MTA and biodentine for primary teeth pulpotomy: a systematic review and meta-analysis of clinical trials. Clin Oral Investig. 2019;23(4):1967–76. https://doi.org/10.1007/s00784-018-2616-6.

45. Fouad W, Abd Al Gawad R. Is Biodentine, as successful as, mineral trioxide aggregate for pulpotomy of primary molars? A split-mouth clinical trial. Tanta Dental Journal. 2019;16(2):115–9. https://doi.org/10.4103/tdj.tdj_35_18.

46. Kusum B, Rakesh K, Richa K. Clinical and radiographical evaluation of mineral trioxide aggregate, biodentine and propolis as pulpotomy medicaments in primary teeth. Restor Dent Endod. 2015;40(4):276–85. https://doi.org/10.5395/rde.2015.40.4.276.

47. Niranjani K, Prasad MG, Vasa AA, Divya G, Thakur MS, Saujanya K. Clinical evaluation of success of primary teeth pulpotomy using mineral trioxide Aggregate((R)), laser and Biodentine(TM) – an in vivo study. J Clin Diagn Res. 2015;9(4):ZC35–7. https://doi.org/10.7860/JCDR/2015/13153.5823.

48. Cuadros-Fernandez C, Lorente Rodriguez AI, Saez-Martinez S, Garcia-Binimelis J, About I, Mercade M. Short-term treatment outcome of pulpotomies in primary molars using mineral trioxide aggregate and Biodentine: a randomized clinical trial. Clin Oral Investig. 2016;20(7):1639–45. https://doi.org/10.1007/s00784-015-1656-4.

49. Togaru H, Muppa R, Srinivas N, Naveen K, Reddy VK, Rebecca VC. Clinical and radiographic evaluation of success of two commercially available pulpotomy agents in primary teeth: an in vivo study. J Contemp Dent Pract. 2016;17(7):557–63.

50. Carti O, Oznurhan F. Evaluation and comparison of mineral trioxide aggregate and biodentine in primary tooth pulpotomy· clinical and radiographic study. Niger J Clin Pract. 2017;20(12):1604–9. https://doi.org/10.4103/1119-3077.196074.

51. Juneja P, Kulkarni S. Clinical and radiographic comparison of biodentine, mineral trioxide aggregate and formocresol as pulpotomy agents in primary molars. Eur Arch Paediatr Dent. 2017;18(4):271–8. https://doi.org/10.1007/s40368-017-0299-3.

52. Celik BN, Mutluay MS, Arikan V, Sari S. The evaluation of MTA and Biodentine as a pulpotomy materials for carious exposures in primary teeth. Clin Oral Investig. 2019;23(2):661–6. https://doi.org/10.1007/s00784-018-2472-4.

53. Percinoto C, de Castro AM, Pinto LM. Clinical and radiographic evaluation of pulpotomies employing calcium hydroxide and trioxide mineral aggregate. Gen Dent. 2006;54(4):258–61.

54. Sonmez D, Duruturk L. Success rate of calcium hydroxide pulpotomy in primary molars restored with amalgam and stainless steel crowns. Br Dent J. 2010;208(9):E18, discussion 408–9. https://doi.org/10.1038/sj.bdj.2010.446.

55. Croll TP, Killian CM. Zinc oxide-eugenol pulpotomy and stainless steel crown restoration of a primary molar. Quintessence Int. 1992;23(6):383–8.

56. Camilleri J. Staining potential of Neo MTA Plus, MTA Plus, and Biodentine used for pulpotomy procedures. J Endod. 2015;41(7):1139–45. https://doi.org/10.1016/j.joen.2015.02.032.

57. Innes NP, Frencken JE, Schwendicke F. Don't know, can't do, won't change: barriers to moving knowledge to action in managing the carious lesion. J Dent Res. 2016;95(5):485–6. https://doi.org/10.1177/0022034516638512.

58. Whitworth JM, Myers PM, Smith J, Walls AW, McCabe JF. Endodontic complications after plastic restorations in general practice. Int Endod J. 2005;38(6):409–16. https://doi.org/10.1111/j.1365-2591.2005.00962.x.

59. Schwendicke F, Al-Abdi A, Pascual Moscardo A, Ferrando Cascales A, Sauro S. Remineralization effects of conventional and experimental ion-releasing materials in chemically or bacterially-induced dentin caries lesions. Dent Mater. 2019;35(5):772–9. https://doi.org/10.1016/j.dental.2019.02.021.

60. Koubi S, Elmerini H, Koubi G, Tassery H, Camps J. Quantitative evaluation by glucose diffusion of microleakage in aged calcium silicate-based open-sandwich restorations. Int J Dent. 2012;2012:105863. https://doi.org/10.1155/2012/105863.

61. Schmidt A, Schafer E, Dammaschke T. Shear bond strength of lining materials to calcium-silicate cements at different time intervals. J Adhes Dent. 2017;19(2):129–35. https://doi.org/10.3290/j.jad.a38100.

62. de Blanco LP. Treatment of crown fractures with pulp exposure. Oral Surg Oral Med Oral Pathol Oral Radiol Endod. 1996;82(5):564–8. https://doi.org/10.1016/s1079-2104(96)80204-6.

63. Ojeda-Gutierrez F, Martinez-Marquez B, Arteaga-Larios S, Ruiz-Rodriguez MS, Pozos-Guillen A. Management and followup of complicated crown fractures in young patients treated with partial pulpotomy. Case Rep Dent. 2013;2013:597563. https://doi.org/10.1155/2013/597563.

64. Shabahang S. Treatment options: apexogenesis and apexification. J Endod. 2013;39(3 Suppl):S26–9. https://doi.org/10.1016/j.joen.2012.11.046.

65. Guideline on pulp therapy for primary and immature permanent teeth. Pediatr Dent. 2016;38(6):280–8.

66. Karabucak B, Li D, Lim J, Iqbal M. Vital pulp therapy with mineral trioxide aggregate. Dent Traumatol. 2005;21(4):240–3. https://doi.org/10.1111/j.1600-9657.2005.00306.x.

67. Simon SR, Tomson PL, Berdal A. Regenerative endodontics: regeneration or repair? J Endod. 2014;40(4 Suppl):S70–5. https://doi.org/10.1016/j.joen.2014.01.024.

Printed in the United States
by Baker & Taylor Publisher Services